Preord
By Death

Errol Edward França Hewitt

chipmunkapublishing
the mental health publisher

Published by
Chipmunkapublishing
United Kingdom

http://www.chipmunkapublishing.com

Copyright © 2016 Errol Edward França Hewitt
Artwork by Susie Hawkins

ISBN   978-1-78382-084-9

PREFACE:

Adorn a crown of virtue surrounded by the night,
a breath of life giving hushes is not without the light.
My soul is violet black in neon, with wings upon despair,
a mist of curls entrances, uplifts a kiss in prayer.
My lady, you will be, above the jasmine's shade,
ivory flowers of beauty, depart all doubts were made.

Errol Edward França Hewitt

The Lord of Death stood watching over the morning sun, next to him was the imp Faramel, who squinted at the early rays of light. "So, the prophecy speaks of this time and this place?" the little imp said.

"Yes," the Lord replied, "Look over there." He pointed to a house which lay on the hill. "This is where the child is going to be born."

They made their way along the dirt path past hedges and fields travelling on a thin mist that was cloud-like, though not as high up, they were inches off the ground. A candle flame could be seen through the top window and the sound of a baby crying out cut through the air, coming from within. The mist rose up so the Lord and the imp could see in. A mother held her baby which was wrapped in a soft blanket and she kissed the newborn's head as a man sat on the bed next to his eldest child and spoke of blessings from the creator for giving them a healthy baby boy. The man thought he heard a sound by the window so he turned around, but nothing was there except he heard a strange whispering as if the wind was trying to speak. He stood up and opened the window wide to let in the cool air, looking at the new light of day and the tint of shade brightening.

Ten years later.

A tree, gnarled and withered, held a wooden shack which was called the *spiders' house* for there were many a spider which could be found within scurrying around. Tinina, was the youngest and she feared going into the tree house because of the spiders. The eldest, Martiv, had put candles in there and would sometimes hoist the rope ladder up so Dorian his younger brother could not climb up. But, Dorian was as nimble as an ant and found foot holes and things to grab onto so he could pull himself up the tree and enter the *spiders' house*, for there was no lock on the door. Inside, there was a book of poems that Dorian had been given a while ago by his uncle. The book was said to have been written by a priest who had changed into a dove and had flown to heaven, but Dorian was sceptical of such notions and thought that the writing was all about nature and angels. Martiv, was burning tobacco in a pipe which he had taken from the shelf of the living room, where their father kept it.

"You will sure get a beating if our dad finds his pipe missing," Dorian said in warning.

"Do you want a puff or not?" Martiv said in a manner of someone who has the power but doesn't want to part with it.

"No thanks," Dorian said and lifted up a cloth so he could look out of the window. Down below he saw Tinina on a swing and just in the distance, where the wood was, a creature of evil was approaching with clawed hands and a bloodthirsty intention. The young girl turned and screamed and before the beast was upon her, Haroman, her father, was charging towards it wielding *steelfang*, his great grandfather's sword. The creature turned and sensed a threat. The blade of the sword struck deep and sprayed blood. Tinina, ran to the safety of the house as her father received a series of cuts from the monster's claws before he thrust *steelfang* into its ribcage and it dropped to the ground dead. The boys were fearful but came down at their father's bidding to make sure that they were okay.

"That was awesome dad. You sure dealt with him," Martiv said in respect.

Haroman, responded, "You do what you have to to protect your family. It's something you will learn in life son."

Dorian, was shaking a little and was thinking what would have happened if their father had not been there. Haroman, gave him a squeeze on the shoulder and said, "Don't be afraid son. There are many other things worse then monsters of the forest."

"Like?" asked Martiv.

"Well, the evil in a man's heart can cause much more destruction than a beast with claws, he can bring down a whole nation," their father looked away and then said, "Back to the house boys, while I go and dispose of the beast's corpse."

The lads ran in to tell their mother what had just happened, but she already knew for she had been watching from the kitchen window and had warned Haroman of the monster.

That evening they sat around the table eating and Martiv was giving description as to his father's heroic battle. Tinina, was terrified at the thought of the beast and was most upset at the mention of it; she ran to her room to cry.

After they had finished eating Haroman went to get his pipe, but could not find it, "Martiv! Have you been smoking my pipe again?"

The boy's face turned to one of worry knowing that in all haste he had forgotten it in the *spiders' house*. His dad came back into the room and said, "You had better go and get it before the punishment I have in store for you gets worse."

Martiv, ran out without a word and climbed the rope ladder and retrieved the pipe. Running back to the house he slowed down and wondered at what the punishment would be. Upon entering, his father had a stern look in his eye as the boy handed him his smoking implement. "Don't let me find it missing again. When you're old enough I will get you your own, but until then don't you dare disobey my instruction," his father tapped the pipe in his hand

and then said, "Tomorrow you will be cleaning out the attic with me while Dorian and your mother will go to the town to get supplies."

"But dad. I wanted to meet up with Tobias. He will be there tomorrow and had promised me to bring a carving knife which his grandfather said I could have."

"Well son. Your punishment will serve me well. And, it is best that you learn to obey me. I only have your interests at heart."

Martiv, turned away from his father in mid sentence and stormed off up to his room slamming the door. Haroman, thought he was being hard on the boy for after all he was nearly fifteen and when he was a boy he had tested his father's temper. Sighing, he went out of the house and filled his pipe, lighting it and drawing in smoke.

The next day when Dorian, his sister and mother, went to the town, Haroman asked Brina, his wife, to speak to Tobias about the knife, for their father wanted to show Martiv that he would be rewarded for his help.

At the town there were many tradesmen. Tables lay adorned with trinkets and tools. Also, there were the sounds of chickens squawking, and doves cooing. Dorian, noticed a soft feathery owl perching on a rod with a small chain attached to its leg. He looked at it and the owl turned its head to settled its wide eyed gaze upon the lad. "This way," his mother said as the boy was transfixed to the mottled owl. His mother led him by the hand up to a grain merchant. The man weighed some pumpkin seeds and *mosin* grain which was used to make a spicy bread and requested seven coins. Brina, paid the man and put her just purchased foodstuffs in a sack which hung on her back. They spent about an hour in the market. Dorian, was allowed to roam around with two coins in his pocket, while his mother and sister went to buy olives and fruit.

Looking around he saw a man selling paper books, so he stopped to look at them, but they were too expensive to buy. After a disappointing search for something interesting, he came to a table with jewellery and curios. There was one necklace in particular which stood out. A series of small sea shells with a black shark's tooth, looking closer there was a rune carved into the tooth. He asked the man how much it was and the reply was, "It is for sale at two coins," the man said and picked it up to indicate small shells that belonged to rare creatures called *nilsos*. Dorian, was captivated by it and handed over the necessary money. He turned to see his mother and went over to her in excitement showing her his new buy. "Two coins you said? That's a lot for just some sea shells. Who from?" she enquired.

Dorian, turned to point to the man who sold him the necklace but he was not there and the boy stood confused, looking around.

"He's gone," he said.

"Well, it was your money. I just hope in the future you don't go and waste your money on something that you could have made yourself," she turned away from him and Tinina was eating a sweet apple on a stick, but instead of feeling envious, for he loved sweet treats, he felt the smooth shells in his hand, thinking that it was coin worth spending.

When in the evening Dorian lay there, he had a strange dream of a man sitting on a chair by the sea telling a story of a great shark that had eaten a king who had been swimming in the sea. The king was wearing a scarf of black dye from the seeds of a tree reputed to be the tree of everlasting power. The scarf stained the shark's teeth and the great fish was named Rom of the deep, now long dead, and anyone who found one of the black teeth would be rewarded with a chest of gold from the royal line of Aberisonian.

The next morning the boys had to go to the chapel to help clean it and were rewarded with a coin each. Inside the holy building there was a statue of a saint. The saint was a woman called Ofelia, she had her hands outstretched in front of her in submission as if in the act of asking for mercy, in one hand there was a ring and in the other there was a flower. As the legend has it she was captured by a sea beast that lived in a cave and her children were eaten alive. Ofelia, herself was reputed to have called upon the powers of heaven and a great light shot from the sky and disintegrated the monster and all she had left of her children were a ring that the boy wore on his little finger and a flower that the girl had picked that very same day. Dorian, touched the stone hand of the saint and felt a shiver run through him, before turning away to get on with the work.

In the coolness of the chapel the boys worked hard, scrubbing and wetting cloth to wipe away the dust. It took them the usual three hours to do what was required and upon leaving Dorian took one last look upon the face of the beautiful saint he admired and noticed something strange. Stopping, and going closer to inspect the mystery, for there was something odd. Looking closer he noticed that the woman was bleeding from her eyes. Crimson tears rolled down her stone face and into her hands. "Martiv! Come here," the younger of the two shouted.

"What now," the elder said impatiently.

"Look! There's blood running down her face."

Martiv, looked at Ofelia and stood with mouth open, "Why is that happening?" Martiv asked his brother.

"I don't know, but we should inform the priest."

Running in to the back room he led the priest whose name was

Plinimon and showed him the scene that was most intriguing. The holy man stood in shock and asked the boys not to mention it to anyone and made them swear so as not to do so and the boys agreed. Then the man said, "It is the holy day of her children's death, it happens every year and I don't want anyone finding out about it for statues that bleed are very rare and would be taken to what is known as the graveyard of the stones of blood and can be used for evil magic and to cast spells on the dead spirits. So, now you know the importance of the statue."

Dorian, was most fascinated by Ofelia and didn't want her to be taken away so he knew he would keep the promise but did not know if his brother Martiv was as honest with his word as he himself was and cast a suspicious eye in his direction.

After leaving the church Martiv said, "I can't wait to tell dad what happened."

Dorian, frowned and said, "You are under an oath not to tell anyone, remember?"

"We've got to tell dad. He will find it most interesting. It is not every day that a statue bleeds."

Turning to look behind him, Dorian could see no sign of the holy man and shook his head in sadness, "What if dad tells someone and they come and take the statue away to cast evil spells?"

Martiv, didn't really hear him for he was caught up in his own thoughts.

At the *castle of fateful night* there was a gathering of the masters. They stood around a blazing fire of green situated in a metallic red chalice, which held a picture of a boy, the boy was Dorian. "It seems that this boy is destined to be one of our servants," master Quintok said raising his hand to his ear and giving it a rub.

Master Shein then spoke saying, "Indeed, the green fires of selection never reveal what is not to be, but it is the wish of higher powers."

"Then, we must find him," master Onis said, "And, the others that have been selected for our tutelage must also be located. So, we will send the guardians to find them."

"I agree," master Quintok said, "All in favour raise their hands."

All held their hands up except master Silvo, he had a sense of the boy Dorian. "Are you not in favour?" asked master Onis.

"There is something about the boy, he doesn't seem noble. He looks weak and afraid," Silvo said tapping his staff with a finger.

"The fire of selection has not been known to be wrong before. You must acccept the decision," master Onis said with a frown, his long white beard showing his age, yet also his wisdom.

The masters left the room and being night, went to their rooms to retire for the evening. As master Quintok and Onis walked the corridors they talked a little and decided to send the guardians the next day to find the children who were to become pupils and servants of the Lord of Death who was the overseer of the castle, above the masters, but also had more responsibility with things that only a lord could be trusted with.

The next day at the castle all were up at sunrise as the bell tolled loudly and all the residents gathered by the waterfall of cold snow, where there was a cloud which dropped snow and as it fell turned to icy water cleaning and vitalizing the bathers in a room with a great depression so the water could build up and drain away. After the cleanse twenty one of the older men and six of the women, dressed in pure white cloaks, mounted their horses, these were the guardians, knowing magic and skill they went into the world to search for the chosen.

The Lord of Death sat on his throne in the room of Holy Immortal. He had a crown of upturned skulls around his skeletal head and with bony fingers played with a rosary, his jet black cloak around his shoulders. Contemplating the search of the children and the prophecy. Faramel, the imp came limping in, having a bad leg, and addressed him as lord and said, "They are on their way. It may take several months, if not years to find the chosen," he said bowing, "And here is what you requested." The imp handed the lord a bag the size of a fist and the lord took it and the fire in his eye sockets flickered briefly. "Thank you Faramel, you have served me well."
The imp smiled, turned, and walked limping out of the room leaving the lord to his own thoughts.

It was a new day and Dorian was studying with his mother how to spell certain words with a test. "It is expedient to learn to spell correctly, for it may get you good work in the future, " his mother said as the boy struggled.
"I know mom, but Martiv is learning sword play. It seems more fun."
"There is a time for fighting and a time for thinking. You know that sometimes it is best to avoid violence. Using your head can get you out of all sorts of trouble. It is best to think first son."
Dorian, let out a sigh for he knew his mother was right. It made sense what she said, and he always had respect for her.
Scribbling away on paper he wrote a piece about a magic rabbit that stole eggs from chickens and painted them, only to return them to the chickens' nests. His mother always liked his imagination and encouraged him to write even though it was all made up.
After an hour the boy was rewarded with hot milk and honey, which

he sipped at and gazed out the window where the tree house was. Martiv, came in panting with sweat pouring off of him and a small cut on his arm where his father had sliced him with a wooden sword which was sharp enough to make a wound. Brina, creased her forehead in stress, "You shouldn't be so hard on the boy Haroman."

"He's got to learn to keep his guard up. It's no use playing soft. You know when danger strikes there is no time to be weak, it could get him killed," their father grinned and Martiv didn't seem to mind that his dad was strict, it just meant that he had to be serious and learn the art of fighting. "The more real the better," Martiv said grinning like his father.

"Well, get cleaned up and lunch will be served in a few minutes, so be quick," the children's mother added a dressing to the salad and sliced some carrot bread. Tinina, looked up at her mother and said, "Nearly finished with the scarf." The young girl had been sitting on a bean cushion knitting a very colourful scarf that had taken her over three months to complete. Dorian, picked up all the paper, ink and quill, stuffing it all into a space in the cupboard out of the way. Sitting at the table he scratched at a bit of dried leek still on his fork which didn't come off when it was washed. His father soon came in with Martiv behind and sat at the table. Tinina, refused to budge until she finished the last line of the scarf and then joined them at the table picking up a piece of bread and dipping it in a buttery sauce.

There was talk of money at the table as Haroman said he was now earning more coin by playing the singulet, an interesting instrument with strings which was played with a bow and made pleasant resonant tones. "The royal hall of the prince has expressed an interest in our trio and has instructed that the choir accompany us, to the delight of his sister Linianne. Our first performance will be in two days. We will be rehearsing here tonight," Haroman bit into a chunk of cheese and Brina said, "That is good news. Especially being able to get a good wage for doing something that you always had a passion doing."

"Yes, you know well that music was my thing since childhood," he said as he prodded at a piece of tomato with his fork.

The rest of the day went by and Dorian had read several chapters of a book on the woodlands. His sister had finished the scarf and wrapped it around her neck prancing about like a fairy admiring herself in the mirror. Martiv, had a few more cuts on his knuckles and Haroman his father had a small gash on his leg where the boy caught him off guard, his dad praised his trickery and patted him on the shoulder saying, "Well, my son. Now you know that your wits and skill can be of use. If you use that sort of cunning against a

11

wood troll you might just slay the creature."

Martiv, broke into a broad smile and said, "Only if the troll isn't as fast as you dad."

"Yes, they are known to be quite slow, but beware their strength is beyond mine. It would take a good focused stroke of the sword to fell one."

The children went to bed for it was late. The choir arrived and their rehearsal was heart warming and exuded a power that was reverent of a higher realm. Brina, sat by the roaring fire with a mug of honey wine and Haroman, when the musicians had gone, left the warmth of the room to sit on a wooden chair, made by his own hands, outside in the cool air. He lit his pipe and puffed away, thinking of the music he had just performed, when he could make out a figure coming along the path on horseback. Squinting his eyes to see better the rider came near and stopped in front of him, "Hello stranger," Haroman said, unsure of who the person was.

"Greetings," the horseman said. "I am in search of a boy named Dorian. I was told that he is your son, is he not?" the man on the horse dismounted and walked over.

"What is this about?" questioned the boy's father.

"My name is Slonic and I am from the *castle of fateful night* and looking for children that are required to serve there. They have been chosen by the emerald fires for the position and are greatly honoured to be chosen," the man offered his hand to Haroman in an act of friendship. The father clasped Slonic's hand, shaking it firmly. "Come inside and we will talk."

The fire was ablaze in the living room and Brina, looked up to see the stranger Slonic. She looked uncertain for a moment until her eyes fell on the crest of the *castle of fateful night* which was a night owl, wearing spectacles; reading an open book, made as a brooch, then she looked respectful. Haroman, introduced the man to his wife and offered him a drink which he accepted. The three sat around the fire talking about the situation. Slonic, sipped a bit of the brew then said, "Yes, it is important that Dorian attends to this request for he will be taught the ancient language of Hermosti and trained in duties that are fitting. He will be taught all the good qualities that one would expect from a child and will be allowed to leave the grounds once a year for twelve days to be with you, though letters can be exchanged on a regular basis. And, of course there will be an income"

Brina was fascinated by all the talk and although reluctant to send off her son she felt it would be for the best. The reputation of the *castle of fateful night* was known for thousands of miles around.

Haroman, thought it was a good plan, but said, "We will need some time to think about this proposal. Maybe a few days."

"Of course," Slonic said.

"You are welcome to stay for a while if you have nowhere else," offered Brina.

"Thank you, it would be most accommodating to stay here. I thought to wrap myself in a blanket under a hedge," Slonic laughed, and the other two also.

Brina, showed the weary man to a room that was for guests and he thanked her. She then said, "Have you eaten?"

"Not for many hours."

"Well, I will bring you up some bread and cheese in a moment," she walked out of the room and he placed his pack next to the bed and pulled out a small book which he began writing in. Soon enough, Brina appeared with a plate of food and left him to eat and get some sleep.

That night Slonic pulled out a crystal and sprinkled a pinchful of dust upon it. Immediately, a picture formed of master Quintok. "I have found the boy Dorian."

"Good," came the reply from the picture that emanated from the gem.

"I think he will be coming with me to the castle within a few days. His parents showed respect for us and our teachings, so there is hope," Slonic scratched his leg and the voice of the master spoke, "Keep careful watch over this one. The lord himself requests it."

"You know I will put my life first if need be," Slonic said with no fear in his voice.

"Let us hope it doesn't come to that," the master waved a hand and the vision was gone. Slonic, lay back in the bed grateful that he was within the confines of a building, and warm.

When the sun was rising and the air was cool Slonic was downstairs sitting just outside on a rug, carving a figure in a piece of wood, which is what he did to pass the time. He used a small knife with a curved end and after a few hours he had completed an image of an elf with pointed ears and a bow in hand. The woodcarving had an exact likeness to Ornmapruviel a female of the elven kind who Slonic had once encountered and couldn't forget. To him she was the most beautiful of all and he longed that their paths would cross again.

There could be heard a noise from within and soon enough Haroman came out and nodded in courtesy and lit his pipe. "It is a fine morning," he remarked and the guardian flicked closed his knife and agreed saying, "Yes, there is freshness in the air."

Brina, called out to them asking if they wanted a brew of *oioip* a herbal plant used in hot drinks familiar in this locality for its strong flavour. The two men answered back in favour of the beverage.

When Haroman had finished his pipe they went in and there were three mugs on the table, steaming. "I'll call the children down in a moment," Brina said. Tinina's soft footsteps could be heard coming down the stairs and she walked up to her mother with a kiss. "You're up early," Brina remarked.

"Yes, I heard you talking," came the meek reply.

"I will make you some fried bread with herbs," her mother said and began busying herself.

Slonic, had left the wooden figurine on the table and Tinina picked it up smoothing the surface of the elf. "What is it?" enquired the girl.

The guardian, Slonic looked up and said, "That is an elf of the far distant forest of Iunin."

"Oh," the girl said and put it down. Tinina, was wearing the scarf which she had knitted and she flung an extra coil around her neck for she felt cold. Her mother was soon done with the fried bread with herbs and Tinina began to eat rather slowly.

The frying pan was soon sizzling away with sausages, other meats, beans and eggs. The three adults were eating their breakfast when Dorian came down the stairs and sat down on a cushion next to the rocking chair. "Good morning son," his father said.

The reply was slow to come but the boy eventually said, "Good morning."

Slonic, looked at Dorian and wondered what the boy's childhood was like here. It was a good place to grow, with caring parents and a safe house in which to pass the time. "Have you given any thought to the boy's future," the guardian asked of the parents.

"Yes, we were up for hours last night discussing your proposal. We have decided to let him go to the castle, for it is a once in a lifetime opportunity," Brina had spoken for both herself and her husband.

"It is wise that he should be taught our ways," Slonic said.

Haroman, then said, "Yes, I will come with you to the *castle of fateful night* to make sure he reaches there safely."

"He will be safe in my hands," Slonic reassured, but Haroman insisted that it would put his mind at ease to know for sure, for they would not hear from the boy in a while until he had settled in.

"Of course," the guardian said thinking that it must be a hard decision to let a loved one go off into the world and at such a young age.

The three travellers were on horseback, making their way through the woods. Dappled sunlight lit up scenes of wildflowers and hundreds of small flies the size of mustard seeds looked like dust in the air. There was a crack in the silence and Haroman spun around to see a lone goblin with a bow. The goblinoid looked stunned as if it had be smoking the infamous *crumbly mud*, which was made from a dried plant and was known to send one's mind into space. Then, the goblin introduced himself as Glom. Dorian, who had stopped and turned said, "What brings you out in these woods?"

The goblin snorted and then said, "Well, I was looking for my brother Phlom, but I've lost his trail."

Haroman, deciding the goblin was off his head, said, "You know any other traveller would have cut your head off by now. Don't you fear death?"

Sighing, the goblin whimpered about having lost his mother by the sword. Dorian, felt sorry for him, but Slonic said, "We should really be moving. This could be a trap," he whispered.

"Sorry, can't help," Haroman said turning his horse and Dorian doing the same. The goblin muttered something and stood there, pulled out a pipe and filled it with *crumbly mud*; lit it. A backwards glance from the boy's father confirmed his suspicions. Slonic, led the way and as night was enshrouding he said, "There is a tavern for wayward travellers up ahead."

Haroman, knew of this and said, "It will be a welcoming sight, for spending so long in saddle."

Up ahead, after another hour of riding, were several small buildings, including a tavern with a sign painted of a bear and wolf. Within the hour they had eaten and retired to a room with three beds. On the table, in the room, was a book of pictures. All of them were hand painted and Slonic thought that someone had left it there by mistake. Flicking through the pages, Dorian saw depictions of gargoyles and stone work. He assumed that it must belong to a stone mason. His father said to the boy, "Be good and take the book down to the barman and say that it was left in our room."

Dorian, after he had finished looking at the finely illustrated work and admiring it, took it down the stairs. Approaching the barman he held the book out and explained that it was found in their room. The man looked through it and said, "The travellers have been gone now for over two weeks. You can keep it."

Thrilled, Dorian tucked the small book into his pocket and returned upstairs to his father and Slonic. That night it was quiet and they all slept without incident. As Dorian lay there he thought of the future and what it would be like at the castle. He wondered if he would make new friends and what the food would be like. Eventually, he dropped off to sleep.

In the first morning's light Slonic was up and went for a walk. He returned an hour later and the boy with his father were both awake and eating cereal on a bench inside. "Good day," said the young maiden, who was carrying some breakfast for an elderly couple with fine clothes sitting by the fire that was burning. Slonic, nodded and proceeded to sit down next to Haroman.

"It is still several days journey to the castle," Slonic said.

"I've never seen it. Just heard stories," came the reply of Haroman.

"It is a place of great spirituality. And also learning."

Dorian then said, "Will I learn magic?"

Slonic, knew that many a child would have liked to learn the arts of spellcasting and for some it was instructed, but he was cautious with his reply so as not to get the boy's hopes up, and said, "Some learn the art, but not all. We all have a responsibility to the Lord of Death and our talents are dispersed in our students so that each one of us will learn something in great detail so as to be of assistance."

Dorian shrugged not knowing if he would be chosen to learn magic, but he was excited about it all for it seemed already like a few footsteps on the path of a great journey had begun.

The Lord of Death was sitting on his throne with a glass of fizzy lemonade on a side table and he reached for the remote control, clicked a button and a wide screen emerged from the floor. Another few clicks and a picture appeared of a man being put to death. He turned the channel and there was a woman being burnt alive. So, he changed the picture again and there was an old man with a grey beard, tied up and taking a beating. At the bottom of the screen there were numbers, according to how long the victim had left to live. The man had six minutes till his death and the lord stood up, reached for his walking stick and tapped his *mino* stone ring saying, "Take me to 9284." Then a cloud surrounded him and he was zoomed to the location of the man being beaten.

The Lord of Death stood there watching the thugs do the man over and within a few minutes the old man's spirit left his body and death said, "Welcome to the immortal."

"Where am I?" the man enquired, and then looked down at his dead body which the louts were still kicking, they stopped and walked off laughing.

"Am I dead?" the man said.

"You have passed on. But, still you live," replied the lord.

The man looked around him and said, "So, where do I go now."

"You go to be judged," the lord said. "In a few moments... Oh here they are, late as usual."

A horde of angel mice descended, flapping their wings, and wrapped the spirit of the man with cords of invisible restraint, lifting him up and leading him away to be judged. The man did not struggle and floated away. Death, then sighed and thought, 'Another sad departure.'

Returning to the castle via the summoning of the magic of the ring, he sat back on his throne and Faramel arrived with a packet of crisps and some biscuits. "Thank you Faramel," the lord said, then pulling out a music console from under the throne, slid a disk of corkscrew blues in and sat back listening to slide guitar, feeling a little depressed. After about half an hour he scratched his skull with a bony finger and reached into his pocket on his cloak clasping a small brown plastic bottle. On the label it said, "Anti depressants, take when needed." So, the lord, feeling an unending gloom tapped two tablets onto his palm and threw the tablets into his mouth with a satisfying sigh he returned the bottle to his pocket.

Riding over a rise in the ground the three travellers continued. It was their forth day on the road and the previous night they had spent in the open with the sounds of creatures in the night. It was a sunny day with sometimes cloud obscuring the sun making it a little cool. They were nearly out of the forest when a cloud of stinging insects descended upon them. Dorian, was bitten three times and Slonic twice. Haroman, the boy's father suffered several stings of venom and cursed the little creatures. When the insects had passed Slonic presented them with a cream which they applied to their sores. "Where did you get this from?" asked Haroman.
"Well, I had the same trouble on the way to find your son. I met a herbalist who travelled with me. In exchange for my sword and food, he gave me the medicine, for we were assaulted in the same fashion."
The cooling sensation of the cream was relaxing and the effects immediate, much to the pleasure of the trio. The uncomfortable feeling of pain soon turned to an irritating itch and was eventually dulled enough not to occupy the mind. Continuing along the well worn mud track the way ahead suddenly took to a rise and the riders kept up the pace and were soon looking down on fields of grain and a river to the east flowed across where a bridge was erected in grey stone. Upon reaching the bridge there was a small wooden hut which was deserted. "I paid coin to cross this way," Slonic said.
"I wonder what has happened to the toll keeper?" Haroman voiced what the three were thinking.
"Maybe, he's gone to get some food," the boy said.
"That's a possibility," Slonic said, and then peered in and saw the man who he had previously seen alive, now lying dead with a crossbow bolt through his chest. "Let's carry on," the guardian said, not wishing to draw attention to the dead man, for it was an ill omen.
Their horses made sounds of hooves on stone as they crossed the bridge and Dorian looked over at the waters which were flowing

where he saw several fish and wished that he could stop and catch one.

A group of several houses came into view and soon enough a small village presented itself with a sign stating the name, Millvon. "I know from experience that we can take lodging at the Farmer's Crop, a local guest house. Of course, I will pay," said Slonic.

Haroman, felt that the guardian was a good man and followed as he led them upto an old building with troughs by the entrance where they tied the horses. Inside the cool interior was welcoming with painted walls and an old plough in the corner with bundles of straw figures arranged so they looked like they were working with scythes. There were a few customers within and some small children playing with dice. Slonic, went up to the owner and started talking to him as Haroman and Dorian sat by the window where there were freshly cut flowers in a vase. "So, are you excited then, about all this?" the father asked his son.

"Yes. I am wondering what it would be like at the castle and what duties will be required of me." The boy rubbed a leaf on the stalk of a flower and then said, "Will you and mum miss me?"

"Of course son. It was not a light decision. But it is the right thing to do," Haroman looked into the boy's eyes and then said, "You will do us proud."

The boy looked away and felt a bit sad. Slonic, soon came over and said we have a room for the night, showing them the key with a number 9 on it. "I'm tired," Dorian said and Haroman suggested that they went to the room. Slonic, decided to go for a walk first and informed them that supper was in an hour.

In the room there was a picture of a mighty warrior fighting hordes of skeletons in battle with the undead. Haroman, pointed out to his son that it was a real war when an evil necromancer had summoned the army of the sleeping dead and caused many deaths in the war. "I think the warrior's name is Illume and he was also a priest," Haroman studied the painting before pulling out a flask of water and taking a gulp.

Dorian, was quite fascinated by this and slumped down on the bed to contemplate one man fighting waves of skeletons and how brave he was. An hour passed quickly and the father with son went down to the common room to eat. They were served with fish and boiled potatoes with green beans. Slonic, hadn't returned and it was dark. After the meal Haroman had a strong drink and Dorian a mug of lemon juice which was to his liking. Another hour passed and the guardian entered the hospitable inn. He sat down by Haroman and said, "There are some of my relatives buried here in the grounds of the village's only church. Just had to pay my respects."

Haroman, completely understood and gave a grave nod of his

head. "So, where do people go when they die?" asked Dorian.

Slonic, answered by saying, "There are many places a soul may journey beyond this life, but there is a heaven where people go to and they meet their old friends and loved ones."

Dorian, didn't know much about the afterlife but was intrigued, and asked, "Does the Lord of Death kill people?"

"The lord," replied Slonic, "Never has need to kill. He visits people in their last hours. Usually people that have been good and he wants to welcome them to the afterlife."

Haroman, then said, "That's enough questions. I'm sure you'll learn a lot more at the castle. But, these things should not be discussed."

Slonic, understood Haroman's superstitious nature and knew that people were afraid of the Lord of Death because of the grim nature of his duties. A man by the bar started to kick up a fuss and was soon launched out the doorway by the barman, followed by the words, "You will pay or do not darken my doorstep again." The landlord then returned to the counter and grasped a handful of nuts that were in a bowl.

A warm wind blew over them as the three travellers descended a hill into a valley. The wild flowers tilted their sleepy heads and butterflies flitted around, darting from one sweet corolla to another. Up ahead, in the sky circled a tableau of pink tailed flishes, their orange beaks and silvery underside made them distinct from many other birds in the land and Slonic admired the swift formations that they made before plunging to then rise. "Just over the next hill," pointed Slonic, "You will be able to see the great *castle of fateful night*."

It seemed like hours had passed when Dorian finally beheld the magnificent grey walls of the castle and its turrets. The boy felt an overwhelming sense of anticipation, also a little fearful at what his future held. For, he was going to begin a new life away from the loving arms of his mother. A thought went to Martiv his brother and his sister Tinina and how long it would be till they saw each other again. It would be several months, and time always went slow, so he thought that Martiv and his sister would not really change that much.

Before nightfall they were at the entrance of the great castle, its portcullis was raised and the three rode in without question. Leading them to the stables, Slonic removed the saddle off of the horse. A boy and a girl soon came to help and they groomed the animals. Dorian and his father were led to a room where they were instructed to wait. It was getting late and eventually Slonic returned and said, "Come with me. I will show you to your room. You will be sharing with Nolon another boy that is going to begin his

19

apprenticeship here. Upon seeing the room, Haroman thought that his son will be living in luxury with the thick velvet curtains, mahogany beds and an open fire which cast shadows. There were also candles in silver candelabras which illuminated an onyx work table which had several rows of books atop. "This is where you will be doing most of your reading," Slonic gestured with a sweep of his hand over the table. "There is a wardrobe to your left where half the space is yours. Now you can unpack your belongings and meet us down in the great hall for something to eat."

Slonic, led Haroman down the stairs to the hall and upon entering there was a great commotion for there were at least three hundred hungry individuals seated eating heartily.

In his room Dorian found that there wasn't much space for his clothes for Nolon's stuff was taking up much room. Stuffing most of his things in, he hurriedly emptied his bags for he was eager to go and eat. It was a matter of minutes before he was out of the door and heading for some grub.

The main hall was easy to find, his ears led the way for the noise of many mouths echoed. Finding his father he sat down next to him and began to eat a dish of healthy food which had been placed there for him. "This seems like a good place," Haroman said surveying the scene. Dorian, agreed and was eager to make friends. Slonic, tapped him on the shoulder introduced Nolon his room mate. The boy Nolon had a kind complexion with olive green eyes and a warm smile. "Hello," he said, and offered his hand for a hand shake. Dorian shook the boy's hand and said, "I'm Dorian."

"I'm Nolon," the green eyed boy replied.

"Pleased to meet you," came Dorian's timorous response.

"Why don't you go and show Dorian the fencing arena," Slonic said knowing that it was quite a remarkable room with all the banners of the lands there. So, the two new friends went to explore and become better acquainted with one another.

Four cloaked figures left the church that had boarded up windows, for the once stained glass had been broken by youths throwing stones. They walked, one after the other hiding their faces. A cart had drawn up by the gates. A burly looking bald man motioned to the ogre to lift a stone statue off of the back of the cart and he lifted it with apparent ease. One of the cowled figures spoke, "Bring the statue inside through the side entrance. We will lead the way." The ogre carried the statue of Ofelia on his shoulder and blood was dripping down his back which came from the eyes of the stone figure. After the ogre had finished what was required of him they returned back to where the man was waiting with the cart. "Here are the coins," the cultist with the sharp nose handed over a small bag of money and the man who had delivered the stone lady emptied the contents onto his hand to make sure the correct amount was all there. He gave a satisfying nod and then went on his way. The hooded cultists made their way back into the unholy church and admired Ofelia. "This will give us more slaves of the damned, and our army will be formidable," the main spokesman was the only one who could speak, the others had no tongues, for they were cut off to ensure the safety of the dark magic that was used at the command of Zronisk the master of darkness as he had come to be known. Zronisk, the speaker chipped off a segment of the statue and went over to where there were a number of coffins. He opened one up and the stench was gross but he had no sense of smell. He made a spell of *mighty force* and crushed the stone into powder saying, *"By this holy dust infused with the blood of righteousness, I command you awake from your sleep."* The dust was sprinkled onto the dead body and within moments it raised a hand, then its eyes flicked open. The undead creature arose and spoke with a hoarseness, "I need blood."

Zronisk, pulled aside his cloak and offered his arm. The cold teeth of the unholy rotting corpse sank into his arm drawing blood and it feeded. Afterwards, the corpse that was alive said, "What can I do to serve you?"

Zronisk, instructed the undead male to dig up the other graves and said, "Be sure to leave the coffins unopened, I like to see how they lay with my own eyes first."

The creature then went out into the shadows of late afternoon and began to dig with its bare hands, clawing the earth and eating thistles.

"You three," the speaker said to the others, "Go and kill. Bring back fresh meat."

The three black cloaked ones turned as one and marched off out into the evening to search for victims.

It was soon midnight and five coffins had been dug up. The first of the necromantic followers returned with a dead female slung over his shoulder, her throat had been cut. "Did you make sure you were not followed?"

The mute nodded.

"Good," the speaker said.

Another hour passed and the other two followers came in. One had a child with a metal hand, dead.

"Good work," Zronisk said not caring that the child was weak and would not be much use.

The other cultist had two poisoned dogs, with muscles and savage jaws.

"They will add to our strength," the speaker said. He then looked toward the stained glass window which depicted a man being decapitated and with a wave of his hand said, "Take the dead down into the catacombs."

Dorian, awoke soon after the first light and took in his surroundings that were still very unfamiliar to him. He slipped on his clothes and headed down the stairs, leaving his room mate still slumbering. In the great hall there were a trickle of early risers, one being his father. Haroman stood when he saw his son approaching him. "I will be leaving shortly." He unbuckled his belt with the sword *steelfang* in a plain scabbard, placing it on the table he said, "This will protect you if ever you need to use it."

The boy was taken aback for it was a magical weapon and rare. "I will take great care to clean its blade," Dorian said gripping the handle and pulling the sword free to admire the fine workmanship.

"It is a fine blade and will serve you well," Haroman, picked up a crust of bread and took a bite then said, "They will look after you in this place and you should learn a lot. There will come a time when you will need to make a living and the more experience you can get, the greater the reward."

The boy nodded and resheathed the sword. He threw his arms around his father and then Haroman left.

For the first time Dorian felt alone, but there was no fear. Nolon, entered and greeted him, "How is it?"

"Okay."

"Did you have a dream of a man poking a wizard with a stiff snake?"

Dorian, wondered how the other boy knew of his bizarre dream, and Nolon saw the puzzled look and said, "There is a room in this castle were no one goes for it is hidden. In this room there is a tree. The tree has magical properties and affects the dreams of everyone in this castle."

"So, how do we know of what's in the room if no one knows where it is?" Dorian asked.

"Well, as legend goes, the only person who knows it is the lord himself, but it is a closely guarded secret."

"Mysterious," Dorian said and then said, "Let's get some food."

The two boys went up to a serving counter where they piled food upon wooden plates. Dorian fancied toast and boiled eggs, while Nolon had fruit and berry water. They sat next to each other and talked of their families. Nolon, also had a tree house in his garden but it had been dismantled for his younger brother fell out of it once and broke an arm. Their mother was concerned so his dad forbade them to go up in it. Disobeying his dad, Nolon was caught in it so the tree house got taken down and Nolon had no pocket money for two weeks. After they had eaten Nolon offered to take Dorian around some of the grounds where there were many things to see.

When it reached midday a bell rang out as someone pulled on a rope. "We are being summoned to the room of Immortal Heroes. Upon entering the grand room, there were paintings of champions and saints, though Dorian didn't have time to admire them for all eyes were focused on master Onis who had a book in one hand. "Welcome to the *castle of fateful night*," he addressed the new comers. "For some of you this is the first day here. You were chosen from the children of the world to come and learn here. It is a privilege and you must respect our rules. There are twenty seven of the chosen," he swept his gaze around the room and then continued, "There is a piece of paper in front of each of you. We request that you draw a picture and write a short piece about your ambitions, you have thirty minutes."

The chosen, sat at small tables while around them the guardians, some other students and masters watched as the young ones scribbled on the paper before them. Dorian, drew a picture of the *spiders' house* back in his home garden, and then wrote that he would like to learn magic and to be able to cast spells. When the time was up the master Onis tapped a small metal triangle and said, "That will do now." All had finished apart from one boy who continued to write. "Stand," came the order of the master, and all stood. "Make a line," he uttered with friendliness. The twenty seven children formed into a queue. "Now, you will all be picked for a particular line of duty here at the castle. You may become gardeners who study herbology and learn to make potions that cure diseases. Another option is that you will be learning the art of war and trained to use several weapons to fight the evil of the land, also to protect the weak. The final career will be to understand the use of magic and learn to make spells that have a variety of uses. All of these options are just as important as one another and once you have become skilled, be it five years or ten, you will then be sent out into the world to bring order and healing to it," master Onis raised an eyebrow and then pulled a fine yellow cloth from what looked like a huge chalice. "Now, one by one I want you to dip your paper into the liquid within the *basin of changing attitudes* to see what colour it turns to," master Onis stepped aside and each of the chosen ones slipped their paper into the clear water. Then each child withdrew back to their desks. Dorian counted three different colours, there was red, green and purple. His was green. After what seemed like a tense silence master Onis said, "All red papers come forth." Ten boys and two girls came upto him and he said out loud, "You have been chosen for combat." Six of the boys let out sighs of clarified expectations, the others looked disappointed. Then, master Onis said, "All who have green papers stand up and approach." Dorian, rose hoping his would be chosen for magic, but when all the greens were before the master he declared they would be learning herb lore and plant care. Dorian, felt sad, for he had expected to be chosen for spell casting.

The remaining seven, broke into smiles and welcomed the thought that they had been given the opportunity to learn magic, which was a rare occasion. Master Onis then raised his voice to continue with the instruction, "You have all now been given what you will excel at, but there are other duties that is required of you. For instance you all will be taking classes in music, languages, art and writing. There will be four hours in the afternoon on the last day for you to study any given subject, so that you may learn a bit about the other arts. Now, master Quintok will be teaching magic, master Shein will be taking the subject of warfare, and I will lead you chosen for plants and potions. So, each to their master," The two masters which he had introduced for magic and sword craft led their subjects out of the room and to the relevant space to begin introductions of the particular skills.

Master Onis, took the remaining eight students out to the castle grounds to where there was a stone structure with creeping ivy covering the facade. Upon entering, it was cool and there were benches lining work tables. Books were piled on shelves and many jars of interesting mixtures were in rows on a long table. The children sat down and the master picked up a stack of exercise books, handing each person one with a pencil. Then, he said, "We will begin this lesson with writing down our names with a slight description of what we look like, and a drawing, so as to remember one another. Then, we will go for a walk on the grounds where I will show you some of the rare trees and medicinal plants." They each took it in turns to stand up front, present their name and allow time for a brief description. One boy raised his hand and said, "Sir, I don't know how to write."

The master, Onis, instructed the boy to go and find the guardian Jod, "He will teach you the skill of writing. When an hour is up come back here to take part in the lesson.

The Lord of Death was watching the television, deciding which murder was the most gruesome so as to visit the poor victim to invite him or her into the world of the afterlife. There was one particular killing which made the lord angry. A young girl was being drowned for being a witch, for she had a bracelet of blue stones. On this world, death knew that the colour blue was a sign of magic and it was a forbidden colour. The girl had thought that it was pretty and had run away from home, which was a house in a small village.

When she had reached the great city she was captured and beaten; thrown into a cell. The monarch of the city had decreed that all witches be sentenced to drowning, So, here was the young female, as men with rough hands plunged her head into a knee deep stream on the outskirts, where her death would not taint the city. The lord knew she had not long to live and tapped his *mino* ring, reached for his walking stick and said, "320948," immediately he was taken in a cloud of smoke to where the girl was being drowned. He watched as the strong men took her weak life away and her spirit rose when there was no breath in her. She looked at the cowled figure of death and smiled. "So, I must be on the other side," she said.

"You are correct. Now you will join the others in this realm of spirit and you will be judged according to your deeds. But, fear not."

A horde of angel mice came from above and the girl thought them delightful little creatures. They wrapped invisible cords around her wrists and lifted her up into the realm. Death, thought this a sad loss, for the girl was innocent. This made the lord angry and he cursed the evil in man and their laws.

Returning to the *castle of fateful night*, the lord reached for his bottle of pills and downed three, for he was feeling particularly down. He then went behind the throne to where there was a calendar. Searching the dates he pointed a skeletal finger at the 23rd of the month where there was written, "Appointment with psychiatrist, 2pm." He noticed it was clearly written by Faramel's hand, for the little imp would deal with such matters. He hummed to himself before returning to the throne to sit and contemplate the day's events.

During that night's sleep, Dorian dreamt of a mother and father fly, putting their maggot son to bed and reading it a bedtime story. In the morning when he was awoken by the bell gonging, he threw back the covers and quickly dressed. Nolon, had also risen and said, "Did you dream of a maggot?"

Dorian, pulled his shoes on and replied, saying, "Yes, but I can't remember the bedtime story his mother read to him."

"Nor can I. But it was an odd dream."

They both left the room and made their way to the great hall where the students were gathering for breakfast. After selecting toast with jam, boiled eggs and water melon, Dorian sat down, soon followed by Nolon. Suddenly, the noise in the room became much louder as it filled out, and the late risers had entered.

Nolon, had been chosen to study sword play and warfare. He talked much about his first class and said that he got the chance to swing around a two handed sword and, "It was heavier than I thought," he said. "And, a suit of chainmail armour is going to be made for me. Isn't that great? Also, we are going to learn to make our own, so that if need be we may repair our damaged armour. I never thought that it could be so interesting."

Dorian, was excited for his friend, but didn't feel as enthused by his own particular occupation, though there were some interesting things, so he spoke about his line of duty, plants and potions, "Yes, it might seem boring to some, but in a way trees and plants are quite interesting. We were told that they emit a lifeforce and that if we learn to see this energy, then we will better be able to heal. There is a plant called *ecquin* and it has the immediate effect to nullify a posion called *serpent's tongue.* Apparently, the poison causes intense sweating for two hours and then the person breaks out in boils, before dying in agony. So, it is an important counter effect to the poison."

"Interesting," remarked Nolon. "It seems like each different task we undertake, makes us more knowledgeable to the point of being able to save lives, whether are own or another."

"It seems like we are being trained to serve and protect," Dorian pointed out.

"Yes, even though the masters are allowed to walk the other worlds," Nolon said.

Dorian, wondered what his friend could mean, so he asked, "What do you mean by other worlds?"

"Well, as far as I know, the masters are allowed to travel to other worlds to stop evil working its work," Nolon said after hearing a conversation with an elder child.

"So, the masters having completed their training are sent out into the universe to bring peace and order."

"Yes, and the others who don't qualify, are sent into our home world to aid the good cause," Nolon said and scratched at his ankle.

"I've heard that there are other worlds, but thought it a myth," Dorian said, feeling somewhat foolish for not putting his complete trust in his father's words.

"It is no myth," Nolon said, "We will be taught about it at some point I presume."

The bell rang out once again and the students left the main hall to go to their particular lessons. In the company of the others Dorian sat with master Onis going over various names of trees and he took the class out to show them the peculiar characteristics of certain leafy specimens. Near the end of the lesson the master gave each pupil a small seedling and said, "You will all keep this plant for a hundred days, by which time it should have flowered. If you fail to water it on any day, there will not be as many petals on the flowers.

At the end of the allotted time you should have ten flowers, with each corolla containing ten petals. You will be rewarded for your patience if you succeed."

After the midday meal there were studies in linguistics and the difficult alphabet of Hermosti which had forty eight characters. The language was quite eloquent and Dorian took an instant liking to it. They were each given a different poem to translate throughout the course of the week, though they were also helped along by means of a dictionary.

When evening came Dorian was tired and lay on his bed with the lexicon of Hermosti open as he tried to memorize the words which most interested him. Nolon, had a musical instrument with strings on and he practised his chords and finger picking. Every now and again he would stop and complain of difficult manoeuvres. He eventually ceased for several minutes with sore fingers. Dorian was looking forward to his first lesson in the following morning, he had chosen the wind instrument *jol* to learn, and he had already some familiarity with it for his father showed him on a past occasion how to play a tune. Dorian, fell asleep with his clothes on and awoke in the middle of the night and realized, so he got undressed and slept more comfortably.

Faramel, dusted the crown of death which lay on a table. Then he polished the scythe which lay behind the throne, unused. He thought to himself that it was a pity the lord had abandoned it for the walking stick, 'He looked much more the part with the formidable weapon clutched in one hand. Though he is getting old with all the complaining of stiff joints and all..." Faramel, then pulled out a tub of wax and began to add shine to the throne. With circular hand movements, adorning the metallic surface with the thick substance, he wiped it away with a chequered cloth and let out a satisfied breath at his reflection on the gleam. After his duties had been done he went to the bathing room and ran a hot bath which he added *bubblemania*, when full he proceeded to slip into it with the sound of popping bubbles crackling. When the water had begun to cool and it was luke warm, only then did the little imp hop out of it. Then, with a sudden thought he went to the calendar and flipped the page to the next month and wrote, "Faramel's birthday," on the thirteenth. He was going to remind the lord of the special occasion for he wanted him to get a present for him. 'After all,' he thought, 'It only comes round once a year and he always forgets. It's not like he can't afford it, with all that treasure in a box under the throne.' The lord suddenly walked into the room and called out in a booming voice, "Faramel, what are you doing?"

The imp jumped and replied, "Oh, nothing. Just adding another date on the calendar."

"Well, I hope it's nothing too important. I've got a lot of work to do without having to go to see people or attend parties," the lord then sat himself on the throne and leant his walking stick on the side. Faramel, then scribbled out his note for his birthday thinking that it was too much to ask of the busy lord.

Zronisk, had a pale complexion and looked at himself in the mirror thinking that his mother would be proud for she was a witch of the dead, though this had been a secret when he had studied at the *castle of fateful night*. His time at the grand abode of death had been an educational one and he had made few friends. Completing the necessary tests of magic he had become known for his spell of *shocking debilitation*, which made the target immobile and frozen with a soreness. He had used the spell on a fellow student when the lad had found a *feather of secret words*, this allowed anyone who used it as a quill to uncover thoughts of the one thought about when writing. Thus, having taken the feather from the lad for his own use, Zronisk had used it to reveal the mind of the Lord of Death. Though, this was difficult for the lord's mind was usually empty, but he had learnt that the crown was the glory of the lord and that whenever the crown was worn there occurred a state of elevation to the mind of the lord and his thoughts included the whole of creation. So, Zronisk after discovering the secret had elected himself to take the crown for his own purposes.

Looking at his reflection, he imagined the crown sitting snugly on his head and the power of knowing what was passing through the minds of others. His thoughts were one of wonder, and through some reason of his own, he thought that the precious artefact belonged to him for he was above any other living thing. After a few moments the dark master went to the room where he writes. There was a table and the *feather of secret words* was propped in a jar of ink. Picking up the dainty feather he thought of his sister and began to write, he had not seen her in years and wanted to know how her mental composure was. The words came naturally and easily... 'Where is that dreaded dog? If I see him he will be getting a tap on the nose for urinating on my pillow. Oh, there's that key I was looking for. I shouldn't leave it around like that, my treasure should be safe enough though. It's not as if I can't trust my friend. Besides, they don't know of the dried frog I use to cast spells on them. The look on Sarina's face when the curse I put on her came to be. She was covered in boils. She thinks that she's so beautiful. I showed her though.'

Zronisk, laughed at his sister's twisted mind and thought that she was truly a sister to have respect for. Placing the quill back into the pot of ink the master screwed up the paper and with a word turned it to flame, throwing it in the air it was disintegrated before it hit the ground in an explosion of ash. He then stalked out of the room to go to inspect the zombie army he was raising.

Down in the catacombs he entered a room that felt cold and the stench of the decay did not register, for he had no sense of smell. Before him were a dozen rotting corpses animated through the magic of blood stone. They sat there oblivious to their condition and willing to serve. Another cowled figure was stirring a stew of blood and gristle. The other cultist poured out measures of this brew into bowls and offered it to the undead. They drank the contents spilling it down their chins and it ran down onto the floor. The third hooded cultist came in and Zronisk ordered him to go and do some more draining. The figure then collected a tube like apparatus and a bucket, and went into the night to the outskirts of the city to raid the cattle farms to drain the creatures of their blood. He also took the cart so that if he accosted any individual the dead body could be transported back to be used for the benefit of Zronisk and his plans to raise an undead army.

In the first hour of sunlight Dorian played the *jol* and formed some pleasant melodies. Nolon, was awoken by the instrument and instead of being annoyed at being woken up, he lay there and listened. When Dorian was finished and it was time to go to the great hall, Nolon said how airy the *jol* sounded. Then, they both went to breakfast. In the hall it was noisy and busy with the hustle and bustle of life. All the students were engaged in eating and discussing things that they had learnt. Afterwards, when the bell clanged out, they went to their separate callings. Dorian, was once again under the guidance of master Onis, and he had already taught them how to make a healing potion, which they still had to practice till perfection. This lesson, though, Dorian was most keen of ear, for it was about how to tame wild animals and there was a bit of magic involved. The master, Onis, spoke out loud saying, "Now, when you are in fear of your life for a wild horned panther is prowling around you, snarling and looking aggressive, you must speak with a calm voice. Say these words, 'Inni Bakam Dromer." Look at the creature straight in the eye and a small blue light will shine from your forehead, this will distract the creature. The light will reflect in its eyes and have a soothing affect. Once this is done then there is very little chance it will attack. Now, for a demonstration I have a vicious rat that is foaming at the mouth." The master pulled out a scraggly rat from a box and it had a collar with a chain. Securing the chain to a metal rod the nasty rat went for his fingers but the master whipped away his hand just in time.

The maddened creature tried to break the restraint but with no luck. "As you can see, this specimen is completely wild and angry. If you offer it a piece of bread it will go for your finger, for it prefers meat. So, we will try to placate it. Lucy, you first," the master moved aside and the girl came over and tried the spell, but no light shone. Then, Mulin, a boy with neat black hair cropped to ear length tried, but with no success. Dorian, stepped over and felt at ease, he said the words, 'Inni Bakam Dromer,' and to his amazement he felt a warmth on his brow. A blue light shone and the manic rat looked at it, then the creature began to calm down. "Now, offer it some bread," Onis suggested, handing Dorian a pinch of a loaf. The boy took the bread and the rat snatched it from his hand. "Well done Dorian," the master commended. The rest of the next hour was writing about and drawing plants. When the class was nearing the end the teacher Onis addressed the room full of students and said, "As you all know there is a class for all the new students about world to world travel with the master Quintok, there you will learn about other planets and the inhabitants thereof. Also, three students will be chosen to go to one of the other worlds sometime next year. Only the most gifted will be allowed to venture into space so I want you all to try extra hard at your studies if you wish to be the one from this class to be chosen. Dorian, felt hopeful because he had just proved that he was capable of magic with his limited experience. Thinking about the lesson the following day occupied his thoughts for the rest of the day.

When, finally the studying was over and the last instructor gave them information on the language Hermosti, Dorian returned to his room to play some music. After this had pleased him he flicked open a book on Weird Creatures Found on Many Worlds, and began to study in earnest, for he wished to know as much as possible about things he might one day encounter. Nolon, soon joined him and they talked for a while until the bell rang out for supper. "It's the elfling Dri who rings the bell," Nolon said.

"I wondered whose job it was," answered Dorian who had never seen an elfling. "What does he look like?"

Nolon, responded, "You've never seen an elfling? Well, he is short, green; has purple lips and speaks very quickly. I think that describes him accurately enough."

At the first afternoon bell, Dorian had been anticipating the sound for the next class was with the master Quintok and about travelling to other worlds. All of the new students were lined up outside the doorway of the lecture room. He approached with a soft foot for he was against haste and allowed himself the thoughts of speculation. 'What will I learn from this master. I think it will be a learning experience. Maybe I might be chosen for worldly travel...' Dorian stopped his thoughts there as the queue began to shorten as they were admitted into the grey stone building. Within the walls of the structure the room was interesting with a great tapestry adorning one wall. It depicted men with their arms raised to the air and what looked like a ball of fire surrounding the base of a chariot which was in the sky. 'Odd,' thought Dorian.

There was a semi circular seating arrangement and the pupils all sat down on the cherry wood. After about ten minutes master Quintok entered with his cloak billowing behind him, he addressed the class, "Good afternoon all." The voices of the ones to study greeted him and he began his lecture. Dorian was amazed to learn about other planets and how there was technology which was likened to magic, but usually worked at the touch of a button. As the master talked about other planets and the things you would find on them, whether evolution had made progress or if the environment was hostile, this all was relevant. "Also," remarked the master, "Technology has advanced so much that some civilizations have the use of space crafts which enable them to explore the galaxies."

Dorian, was captivated and when it came time for questions he asked, "What does a space ship look like?"

"Good question. I was saving the visuals for the last part of the lesson, so you will have to wait. But, I can tell you that most habitable planets have the raw materials to engineer these remarkable futuristic vehicles."

Dorian, was a bit lost but was looking forward to what the master called visuals. A few more questions and then the lecturer returned to illuminate further the importance of understanding what one may need to know if ever they set foot on a different world.

When more questions were answered the master then turned their attention to the final revelation that he was going to show them. "Please lower the curtains," he requested of several students and the room went dark. The talking ceased and with magic there was shown planets revolving. These celestial spheres were magnified and to the amazement of the spectators there were revealed magnificent buildings. Structures of immense size and complexity. Space crafts zoomed into space and alien races were uncovered as ways of life became clear. Several minutes passed as various modes of living came to light. Then, when the pictures were extinguished master Quintok said, "Now, you will hear several languages, one of them being Hermosti. For the next ten minutes dozens of unfamiliar sounds were unleased, some with eloquence, others harsh and abrupt. Dorian, identified Hermosti, for the voice of the speaker uttered a word that was in his realm of understanding. It was an honour to be able to hear the idioms of other races that were so far away and may never be heard again, Dorian, appreciated the teachings of the masters and wondered if he would be one of the chosen to travel to one of these exotic places.

That evening as Dorian was polishing *steelfang*, his great great grandfather's sword, there was a knock on the door and when Nolon opened it standing there was Faramel the imp and he requested Dorian. Lifting up his head from his work, Dorian arose from the chair and walked to the door. "What can I do for you?" Dorian said.

"My name is Faramel," came the meek response, "And, the Lord of Death requests your presence."

Dorian was speechless, for even some of those who had been here for over a year had not even seen a hint of the great lord himself. "Okay," the boy said turning to look at Nolon's speechless expression.

The imp led the way into the courtyard to where the great building of decay stood with its outer fabric made from a sort of skin that replenished itself every three months, leaving a layer of dust to swirl around the streets within the castle walls. Two guards with swords in scabbards stood erect at the entrance. Faramel, strode upto them, they looked at him and without a word spoken the boy and imp entered the great structure. Within, there was a tiled floor. Paintings of saints were shown, hung on the walls throughout the corridors. The imp paced slowly and led Dorian into a main room then into another hallway where there was a stone mosaic pattern decorating a section of wall. Faramel, with purple lips quivering, mumbled something and tapped several of the little square stones, that made the tableau, at a startling speed, then waited. A few seconds passed then each of the separate stones that made the picture began to spin. The pieces withdrew and a stairway was revealed. Ascending the steps the two took several minutes and Dorian was soon out of breath. Upon reaching the top and walking through a medium sized room, Faramel swung open one of two heavy doors and entered the room of Holy Immortal. Sat on a throne and wearing a crown of upturned skulls, so the teeth curved upwards, was the lord himself. Dorian, felt fearful, but knew that the lord was not evil, though he surrounded himself with death and decay. Nolon, once told him that the lord had to be acquainted with the morbidity of death so as not to go insane, for his line of work was demanding. Dorian, walked slowly towards him and looked about to see rows of skeletons lining the walls. They were of all sizes and races, some were clearly not of this world. "Admiring my

32

collection of bones," came the voice of death as the boy came into hearing range.

Dorian, gulped, then said, "Yes, most unusual."

The lord stood up and walked to him. Pointing at a huge skeletal figure he said, "This one is a greater Ogra, from the vast tundra of Somlis the desert planet."

Boney horns adorned its head and its hands bore spikes of a similar fashion. Dorian, was awed at the sight of something so rare.

"Follow me," the lord said, and the boy was led to a table where there was a Nox board with pieces lined up in circles. "Do you know how to play this game?" the lord asked.

Dorian, was familiar with the game, as his father had taught it to him a couple of years ago. "Yes," was his answer, "But, I'm not very good at it."

"Well, we will sit down and play," the lord said in a baritone voice.

They both sat and the lord said, "You go first."

Dorian, looked at the board and after a few seconds made a move. The Lord of Death spent the next hour ruminating on which piece to move and could tell that the boy was getting fidgety, so he rose up and said, "We will continue this game tomorrow. But for now you can clean my crown of skulls." The lord took off the crown and Faramel appeared with a tub of oil and a cloth. The lord resumed his place on the throne and Faramel said to Dorian, "Be careful not to drop it."

The boy then spent a reasonable amount of time making the crown clean for it had gathered dust and grime over the decades, even though Faramel had cleaned it recently. Sitting on the floor he smelt a flowery scent. Looking around he found the source, under the throne could be seen a small pot with a flower growing in it. Dorian, was amused for the lord was growing petals, leaves and stem in the darkness. The lord noticed the boy's attention and said, "It's a hobby of mine. Growing things." Dorian, didn't ask why but handed the Lord of Death his crown, which he inspected and said, "Thank you. It is much better."

Dorian felt a sense of achievement and Faramel escorted the boy back to his quarters and said, "We will see you tomorrow, as I presume you want to continue the game with our lord?"

"Yes," came Dorian's tired reply, "And, thanks."

The imp then went his way and when Dorian entered his room he was bombarded with questions from Nolon.

The Lord of Death was waiting, with his black hooded cloak pulled over his head, and walking stick leant by the side, in the doctors lounge. The receptionist called out, "Arthur Gimbold. Room 7." A man in his late thirties stood up and walked down the corridor to where room 7 was, he was limping and the lord thought he was going to get a remedy for his ailment. Another name was called out before the lady behind the counter said loudly, "Lord of Death. Room 2." The formidable skeletal form of the lord rose and walked down the hallway to find the room, raising an eyebrow or two from the others waiting. Upon entering a well lit room the psychiatrist, doctor Grongsk a young female goblin, sat with her legs folded and said, "Hello, lord. So what can I do for you then?"

"I don't know. You tell me you're supposed to be the expert," the Lord of Death found a seat, sat down and huffed.

"Well," the goblin said, "What seems to be the problem?"

"It started about a month ago," the lord remembered, "I decided to grow a flower and since then I've been getting bouts of depression.

"You know you've got quite a morbid job. Isn't it to be expected?" the psychiatrist said looking through some of his notes which had been compiled over the time he had been seeing her.

"Yes, but surely a flower is something to be happy about?"

"Well, if it's happiness you're after, why do you do what you do?"

"I was chosen for the role of lord. My family considered it a great honour and it has been my occupation for thousands of years."

"Don't you get bored?" the doctor said frowning.

"No. I find ways to amuse myself."

"Like?"

"Well, I used to breed two tailed *wrots*."

"And this was fun?"

"Yes, but I couldn't help feeling disturbed when they ate each other."

"So, wouldn't it be more appealing to paint or learn a musical instrument?" the female goblin said hoping to spark a sign of creativity.

"I was advised many years ago to never look on beauty, for it was said that in my position it would end in madness. There was something written that I was to surround myself with sorrow and suffering. This, it was said, was to protect me from the perils of the job. I was expected to be frightening and to show no sympathy," the lord sighed and scratched at his leg.

"And you are looking a bit thin," the doctor said concerned. "Have you been eating properly?"

The lord laughed, "Every so often," he said knowing that he didn't necessarily need to eat to survive for his magical nature was self sufficient.

"Well," the goblin doctor said, "We need to get some meat on those bones. I will be referring you to a nutritionist. And, your prescription for anti-depressants will continue."

"Is that all then?" the Lord of Death asked.

"Yes. Give me a call if things get worse."

Leaving the room the lord found his skeletal horse outside and mounted it, before taking to the air and flying back to the *castle of fateful night.*

It was early in the morning and Dorian was walking near a row of trees that lined a pathway to a garden. There were few out this early, but Dorian was restless and had decided to get some fresh air and do some writing and practise the language Hermosti. A little way to the right he saw a young girl about his age and she was sitting on a curved wooden bench with a wand in her hand muttering something he couldn't quite make out. He approached and she stopped her words and looked up at him. Her soft, light brown skin and bright blue eyes instantly made him feel that she was most beautiful. "Hi," Dorian said.

"Uh, hello," came the meek response.

"So, you were chosen for magic?" Dorian said smiling.

"Yes, but I would have preferred to have studied plants," she had a hint of a smile aswell, turning the corner of her lips.

Dorian, was astounded that someone would rather be studying with master Onis in plant lore than magic. "Why?" was his response, for it intrigued him.

"Well, I feel close to nature and I love growing things."

"I would have liked to study magic. You have been given an honourable position, many would have liked the opportunity that you have been given," Dorian, sat down beside her and placed his books on his lap.

"I know, but I'm not complaining. Magic, has an interesting side to it. I mean, um, you can make things levitate, which is what I'm trying to do to that stone on the floor," she pointed her wand at a rough small rock on the ground and waved her hand saying some words. The rock just stayed there unmoving. "I am finding this particular spell difficult," she said. "Sometimes it works and other times it doesn't." She tried again and this time the stone rose up in front of them.

"Well done!" said Dorian totally amazed.

"That's not it," she said, "I have to make it spin aswell." She frowned in concentration and it started spinning. "Now I have to make it shoot out somewhere, maybe over there at that tree."

Dorian, was captivated as the stone sling shotted past the tree. "That was brilliant!" he said.

"Not perfect though," she said. "I am supposed to make it explode before it collides with anything to pass the test."

"That sounds tricky," Dorian said, "But, you are nearly there."

"Yeah, it might take a few more hours till I get the hang of it..."

35

Dorian, opened a book on the ancient language and started to read from it taking notes and correcting mistakes. A thought occurred to him as the girl was using her magic. So, he asked her her name. She replied, "My name is Azul."

"My name is Dorian," he said and they shook hands. He felt that this was the beginning of a friendship that would last and after an hour when Azul had managed to perfect her spell casting with an exploding rock which made Dorian give her a round of applause, she smiling, they walked back to the entrance of the main building to have breakfast. "See you later," she said and wandered inside to eat as Dorian went to his room to put his books away.

In the afternoon, with a pad of plain paper and a pencil in his hands, Dorian sat by the illusion wall, which was in the art room. There were several students there drawing and painting. On the wall was a picture of another world where the trees were silver and the sky a shade of orange. Dorian, was trying to capture the gnarled bark of one of the trees and didn't worry about the background. He thought he was not very good at art but he had a liking for it. After about half and hour he had finished the tree and was quite pleased. Then, he walked out and went to where the fountain was to sit and listen to the water. As he approached he saw Nolon there sitting with a friend talking about music. He sat down and was silent, lost in his thoughts. Nolon, then turned the conversation to Dorian, "So, what have you been up to this afternoon with your free day?"

Dorian, rubbed at a bit of moss that was in between the stones and said, "I've just been drawing a silver tree from the world of Jininakcria. It was most difficult to catch the shining of the sunlight on the bark."

Nolon's friend then admitted, "I find art really boring. My dad says that it takes a lot of patience but it doesn't interest me. So, I would rather be out hunting, which is what I usually did while my sister would spend hours drawing. She is really quite good now."

Nolon then joined in saying, "Art is okay. But I prefer music."

They talked a little bit and then the three went to the magic class that was open to anyone. This was the first time the three had the chance to learn the mystical art of spell casting, so they were alive with anticipation and were intrigued at what to expect.

Stepping through the doorway there was a table with a selection of wands. The young woman who was seated there said, "You must choose a wand for the class."

Dorian, looked at the selection and chose one with a yellow tip which looked like a flame and then went to sit close up to the front so he could hear everything the master Quintok would be saying.

Master Quintok began with holding in front of him an apple and it gradually lifted up and began to unpeel, then it seemed to be cut with an invisible knife into segments which in turn flew into his mouth and he eventually ate the whole thing except the core which was neatly shaped. "I started this lesson with a demonstration of magic, which I think you all know is shrouded in secrecy and ignorance. By showing you some of the skills I have by way of the use of magic by peeling and slicing the apple I hope that you are now aware of some of the things a magic user can do. It takes time to perfect the nature of the craft but as you will learn, it is not inconceivable. The trick with the apple was an example to show you how to manipulate material objects, plus I had a craving for some fruit, so both problems were solved." There were a few outbreaks of laughter, then the master turned to the wall which had a drape of rough green material and waved a hand by it. Immediately words appeared there and he spoke again, "I would like it if at least half of this class would succeed in this short incantation. Umiin Hofi Obu. These words will allow you to execute a magic spell using your wand. It is easier to cast magic through a wand especially if you practise often." He looked around the room at the students and then went over to a chest and opened it. Out popped a yellow head with a long nose, "Meep," was what the creature said and then hopped out. "This," master Quintok said, "Is my little helper. Known as Ulung. She is a native of Jininakcria and likes living in the box." Then, he said a few words to her and handed a small bag into her hands. Ulung, then proceeded to walk around and give each person a small green berry. As she was doing this the master continued, "What I would like you all to do it have in your hand this berry and with a wave of the wand say the words here," he pointed to where the glowing words were on the fabric. The trick is to levitate it from your hand into your mouth. Almost at once the room then came alive with the voices of the students and after the first few minutes several of them had succeeded. Dorian, though, was having difficulty with the spell but much to his surprise the berry lifted up to his mouth and inside. There were a few disgruntled sounds coming from the ones who didn't have success. "Once you have mastered the complexities of spell casting you can make the berry explode in your mouth, quite and experience, though the shock to the back of your throat is amusing." He smiled and said, "This is the first lesson in magic. Next week you are all welcome to return to learn a new spell. But, for now you have other studies that are probably more important than learning neat little tricks." He then walked out knowing if he stayed he would be bombarded with questions from the studious ones, and knowing that it would take a lot of time to explain the

37

things that they all wanted to learn he left without a thought for the hungry magic seekers.

That night Dorian was cleaning the crown of Death and he noticed something strange. There were jewels set in among the eye sockets of the upturned skulls and within each gem there was a small shining light. Though, within three of the jewels there was no light. When Faramel returned Dorian said to him about the lights that were extinguished in the gems. "Yes," Faramel the imp said, "It is a problem."

"What does it mean?" enquired Dorian.

"Well, it has something to do with the nature of the Lord. It is a sign that things are going to get worse for him."

Dorian, wondered what this could mean, but didn't push the imp for any more information because he didn't want to pry too much into affairs that really had nothing to do with him and it seemed that it could be personal. He finished polishing the crown and then waited for Faramel to return. Within an hour the Lord of Death appeared. "Hello," Dorian said.

"Good evening," he replied and sat down on the throne and pulled out a packet of crisps. While Dorian stood there the Lord munched and as he did so he said, "Shall we continue our game of Nox?"

Dorian, looked to where the board and the pieces were where they had played the previous night. "Okay," came his response. It was the Lord's turn to move and as the boy sat there waiting for him to move a piece the lord gave sighs and whispers to himself as if deciding which was the best move. About an hour later nothing had changed and Dorian didn't dare say to him to move a piece. "We will continue this tomorrow," the lord said. At that moment a rat about three feet tall dressed in a shirt with a small jacket and trousers came in and he had a small sword strapped to his side. "Ah, Juiz," the lord said with a hint of seriousness."

"I have returned," the speaking rodent said.

"Did you deal with that unspeakably evil man?"

"Yes, he has been judged," the rat said as his whiskers twitched.

"Good. I will need you again at some point, but for now I will pay you for your work." The Lord whipped out a cheque book and scribbled an amount on it; signed it and handed it over to the rat Juiz who kept a serious face. "It is your usual monthly pay. The world is a better place because of your work," the lord returned the cheque book to a hidden pocket of his cloak. Dorian, wondered about Juiz and what work he was employed to do, then the lord turned to him and said, "Same time tomorrow evening." Faramel then led the boy out and he returned to his chambers.

The very next morning Dorian and Nolon were expected to go to the holy temple of the Virtuous Creator where the students were required to listen to a sermon and to pray. Not all the students had turned up this early for the sun was just rising. Haroman, Dorian's father, had always encouraged the boy to pray because he knew that it was a good thing. A prayer was said for the suffering and afflicted then the priest spoke, "Let me begin with the ways of the Ultimate Corruptor. It is a force, an evil presence which seeks to destroy all virtue. It lurks in each shadow and draws people to commit crimes. It will never rest until goodness is completely corrupted. Some say that it is a solitary being that is purely evil, but the followers of this dark entity claim the title of most corrupt for themselves. It is thought that this malign source is a negative collective energy and being that are the wrong doings of humans. Though, it is known that the dark gods serve no one and that their evil followers pay them homage. These corrupt deities use the dark stream of consciousness to spread diseases and suffering and let us not be fooled, there is only one evil god that is above all the others and he is known by many names that we do not utter, for utterance brings forth his power. To be a servant of the Ultimate Corruptor is to deal out pain and torture and his rewards are unspeakable. Now, our most cherished God of Virtue is kind and wise. He knows our needs and as long as you serve a higher ideal, one to please him and to follow the ways of goodness and virtue, he will bless you with his protection against the Ultimate Corruptor. Now, I will summon an angel so you may see the beauty of the heavenly beings. The priest waved his hands in the air and spoke an incantation. A light shone then grew into the form of an angel. The brightness was unlike any light Dorian had seen before, it was almost blinding and was pure in its whiteness. Before the congregation there was a blissful angel hovering with her wings gently moving. The whole of the people were silent in awe, then the angel sung a song and it was the most divinely inspired music Dorian had ever heard. It seemed to last for about twenty minutes then the angel smiled and vanished. The congregation were totally amazed and the priest was the first to speak, "That was the angel Hosia. She serves the God of Virtue."

Zronisk, the master of darkness, was whispering to himself as he walked around inspecting his undead army. There were now over 40 undead and feeding them was a problem. There were three buckets of dark blood and the zombie boy with the metal hand was lifting up cupfuls of the liquid and offering it to the rotting dead humans that were now living. They drank and spilled the red fluid down their chests. The three followers in black robes watched without an expression and their leader said, "It is nearly time..."

The *uminin* plant that Dorian was to look after was doing well and had sprouted three flowers each with a ring of ten petals. Dorian, touched the soft black stem of the plant and felt a cool sensation like ice without the sting. His eyes moved to the chair where lay the *jol*, its fine craftsmanship admirable. He picked up the musical instrument and sat on a comfortable chair without any arms so as not to make it difficult to play chords. As time passed by his skill, it seemed, was improving and he was careful to execute the notes so they didn't buzz or were muffled. A sheet of paper lay in front of him with the music written, also there were the words of a song penned in red ink in the language of Hermosti. It was a hymn to the great Creator and the blessings endowed to those that follow the path of virtue. Dorian, was still trying to perfect the music and was having particular trouble with a manoeuvre from one chord to another. What kept his interest and energy alive was to complete the song for the music to him was most beautiful and having read the words was looking to singing them with heart. Nolon, came into the room and was humming. "Hi Dor.." he said as he sat at the onyx work table and pulled out a book which had two bookmarks, one for Dorian and the other for him. Flicking through the pages he stopped and pondered on a picture of a mighty warrior with a shining sword doing battle with a monster that looked terrifying. He read a bit more and was almost half way through the volume where Dorian was only about an eighth of the way. It wasn't a race and because it was about Heroes of Legend and it was Nolon's passion it was understandable. Though, the book, which was called Magic and Spellcaster's Way, Dorian was near the final chapter and Nolon himself was still on the introduction.
There was still two hours to go until supper was to be served and Nolon was getting grumblings in his stomach. "Dor.. Let's go to the kitchens and get a sandwich."
Dorian, was also a little hungry and welcomed the idea and the two left and made their way there passing the statue of Lady Imosha who recited a poem in Hermosti as they walked by. Within the kitchen there was a *dragonite*, who was a female and had the features of a dragon but a humanoid form about four feet in height. She, was chopping vegetables as the crew she was in charge of were washing and preparing food for dinner. Her head snapped up at the sound of Nolon clearing his throat to get attention. "Yes," came her deep voice as she threw a handful of sprouts into a pan.
"Well, we were hoping for a snack before supper," came Nolon's gentle yet nervous response.
"Horonimus! Get these two hungry ones some of those pies we

have reserved for the ones who either eat too much or are generally hungry and will stop their grumblings!"

A skinny lad, with green hair dyed pink at the tips, fumbled with a cupboard and withdrew a plate of pies from within. "Take one, and one each only," he said in all seriousness. Nolon, was quick to choose the one which looked big but immediately shrank to half the size when it was in his hands. Horonimus laughed at the disappointed expression on his face and said, "My magic. It serves you right for being greedy."

"I'm not greedy. Just famished," Nolon said in defense.

Dorian, picked one that looked ample enough and the boys left eating the tasty food. "That was a mean trick," remarked Nolon as he shook the crumbs from his shirt. Then noticing an elfling walking towards them he said, "That's Dri, the elfling that rings the bell." As Dri got closer Nolon stopped him and said, "Hello."

The elfling smiled and he had a small clock strapped to his wrist with two silver bells and a small hammer ready to work at a given time. "Hello you," Dri said.

"This is Dorian my room mate. We were talking about who rings the bell when it is time for breakfast."

"Yes, it is me. And, don't complain that it is too loud. Personally, I don't think it is loud enough, with all the late risers becoming more each week," the elfling scratched at the side of his head.

"Are you ever late ringing the bell?" asked Dorian.

"Never," came the reply. "I actually time it to the second in case you are wondering. Sometimes, if I feel daring, I ring it four seconds early, but not too often."

Dorian, laughed. "Well, I am not worried about four seconds. Usually, I am awake by then."

"So you should be," and Dri paused before walking off, saying, "I need to clean the bell. I have approximately one hour and thirty minutes seven seconds before the next ringing and it doesn't sound the same if it hasn't been cleaned." Nolon and Dorian exchanged remarks on the elfling agreeing that he was indeed a unique character and that from what Nolon knew the clock strapped to Dri's wrist was to ring ten minutes before an appointed bell ringing for gatherings in the great hall in case he forgets, "But, he never forgets," remarked Nolon, "It is a well known fact. Apparently, he has remembered to ring the bell with the rope for the last thirty years."

"That long," remarked Dorian.

"Yes. It is said that his father and before that, his grandfather held the position of ringing the bell."

"It runs in the family then," Dorian said with comprehension.

"He is a very amicable character, no one has a bad thing to say about him," Nolon said, "Unlike some other elflings that only get up to mischief in the woods throwing berries and nuts at people." They walked on each eventually going their separate ways

On a comfortable chair, Dorian, was reading from the book of Everlasting Truths, which was given to him by the priest at the holy temple. It was written by many writers and was said to originate from the divine angels that conveyed God's message to the chosen few that served him. These angels were said to whisper into the ears of men the words to be written and therefore a lot of the text was about following virtuous living. He pondered over a few verses and reflected on the words that encouraged prayer saying that when one prays for the suffering of others to be lessened then this helps them, explaining also that if you share in the suffering you will be rewarded at a time unexpected. Dorian, then made a prayer to share in the suffering and so to ease the pain of others that are good hearted. Opening the book to read a little more he learned not to reward evil doers for they will use their gains to hurt and corrupt others. But, it said if they have need for sustenance it is better that they eat and to show goodness towards them so they might learn to be a better person one day. After reading this Dorian placed the book on the table and went for a walk. About an hour later he was feeling a little discomfort as anxiety was creeping upon him. It didn't feel good and he thought it must be the prayer he said. The dust from the building of decay was also swirling around and he suddenly felt that he needed to lie down so he returned to his room. When, lying on his bed he regretted the prayer he said because he felt awful, but soon fell asleep where he dreamed of a family somewhere in a world, they were homeless and starving wandering across a country to reach another province where they sought aid. Looking upon the man and his wife with their two children, a boy and a girl, he saw their unhealthy sunken faces and the sun was scorching down upon them. The youngest, the girl staggered and fell. The family continued on knowing if they stopped they would all die. Then a voice whispered, "With your strength she will rise." The girl got to her feet and stumbled after her family who were a little way ahead and her mother turned and smiled, still with tears in her eyes at the thought of losing another child.
When Dorian awoke he was refreshed but still felt a little bad. A look again at the book of Everlasting Truths around the verses of prayer it mentioned that the divine prayer of suffering was only to be said once a week at the most. Dorian, wondered at the poor family of his dream and wished for the young girl to make it to aid, thinking that he would gladly share in her pain if it would give her the chance to live.

It was 2pm and the heat of the day was most hot. The Lord of Death lay on a reclined deck chair and was sunbathing, on the roof of the *building of decay*, hoping to brown his bones with the sun. Faramel, came up with a tray bearing a jug of lemonade with ice and three glasses. He sat on a cushion and poured the lord a drink and then one for himself. "Expecting someone to join us?" asked the imp.

"Yes, Juiz should be here shortly after he has completed his latest task," the lord spoke and adjusted his sunglasses for they kept slipping down, for he had no ears, just a clean skull with the crown upon it. "Have you ever seen the lake of sun dancing shadows?" the lord asked of the imp.

Faramel, thought this was a bit strange because the lord was not supposed to reflect on beauty, it was bad for his mental health. "No. But I have heard it is a sight to be seen before one parts from this earthly life."

"I would like to go there some time," was the lord's response.

"You know, lord, that you should abstain from what we might call *nice* or otherwise *delightful*."

"I'm tired Faramel. How long have I been lord?"

"At least 130 thousand years. But, you were chosen like the boy Dorian."

"Yes, it seems that he would take my place someday, but it is just a rumour, isn't it?"

"Well, the prophecy says that it will happen, it's more than just a rumour."

The lord laughed and spat a stream of lemonade onto the floor, "I feel strange, and I like it."

"Greetings!" said Juiz the rodent that was much bigger than any rat and more appropriately dressed.

"Hello," the imp said cordially.

Juiz, took the other glass and filled it with lemonade and a few ice cubes seating himself on a plush chair that had been brought up for his person. "What a day it has been. Just one thing after another."

"Anything serious?" asked the imp.

Juiz, took a deep breath, "The morning began with the number 34983290 if I remember correctly. The man who I had to judge was difficult to locate because he is a shapeshifter, which caused a certain amount of misunderstanding. Eventually, I found him in his usual form playing cards with a couple of thugs. He is blind now, but I had to lead him away from the game he was playing by use of an illusory gold coin that rolled along the path, for him to follow, until he was out of their company, for I didn't want to blind the others who, their time will come, but were in effect not to be

43

judged."

"It must be difficult to do the work you do without some form of guilt," the imp said wondering if Juiz felt any remorse.

"Not really," came the reply, "The way I see it is that they deserve far worse for their crimes and it is a pleasure really to make their lives a lot more difficult because in the end they don't deserve to live."

"I suppose it gives them time to think over the wrongs that they have done," the lord said, "And, when I choose a victim for you Juiz, you know I find the most vile criminals for you to judge," the lord took a sip at his drink and smoothed some sun tan lotion on his ribcage.

"Yes," said Faramel. "Let's hope that they will learn something from their horrid endeavours by being in the darkness of sightlessness."

"Let's not talk about it shall we, it is a bit disturbing," the lord said.

The imp looked a bit shocked and Juiz said, "Disturbing! I remember stories of you taking a bath with feline corpses just to get an odour of decay about you, and not to mention the very building you spend most of your time in rots away and dusts the whole of the castle's grounds with its decadence."

"Oh, yes. Something must be done about that. I am finding myself choking on the wind of late," the lord made an involuntary cough and threw an ice cube over the edge of the tower with no concern if it might impact on anyone.

The three continued their conversation for an hour more; Juiz and Faramel grew more and more to suspect something had changed with the Lord of Death but didn't mention it until they left and had a short conversation in another room coming to the conclusion that all the jewels for the crown will have to be replaced.

On this day many of the students had to attend a lecture by one of the masters. It was considered essential for reasons that would become apparent. Dorian, Nolon and a few others went to the spacious room where the lesson was to be and Azul, with her soft brown skin, green eyelashes and bright blue eyes sat next to Dorian, "Hi," she said.

"Hello, this is going to be interesting," Dorian said, not really knowing exactly what the talk was about but was certain it would be most expedient. Azul, pulled out a note book and a pen, "I had better take notes. I find it easier to take in if I'm jotting down stuff at the same time."

"I find it difficult to write and hear everything that is being spoken at the same time," Dorian said and looked over to where the master had just walked in with his long white beard swaying until he came to a stand still. Master Onis raised his hand and waited for his pupils to come to a silence; when all was quiet, being against haste, he kept them in expectation for a good minute. Then he began to speak, "This lesson is of great importance and will take some time to digest. I will begin with the concept of the Ultimate Corruptor. It is a force which is completely evil and lurks in every shadow and is a speck of darkness, this creates a painful emotion. Then, there is an opposite, a Virtue Manifest which is a supreme perfection and is not in all things but is like a star which creates a positive emotion. These two forces are what can make us good or evil in character, most of the time, people in general, possess a mixture of these qualities, it just depends on the individual. The Ultimate Corruptor urges us to do bad things and wants to destroy all virtue. While, if we have any virtue in us we will fight these temptations and struggle. The evil force wants complete corruption and therefore the spark of virtue is threatened. Where there is light there you will find virtue, for light itself is a good thing.

Now, let's move on to the qualities of our nature. There are ten main qualities, five corruptions and five virtues. So, we may have a mixture of these principles at work in us and that makes us who we are, our struggles, failures and successes. We will start by explaining that disturbing force of corruption, for I want you all to be well aware of the nature that this may bring and the threats that it can incur.

Darkness, brings forth negative emotions, be it: hate, fear, lust, envy or anger. They affect our thoughts and are devious sensations which sometimes we may not be aware of unless we are taught how to recognize them. You can train yourself to recognize the negativity by using your awareness to see the reaction you get to your emotions. If you feel any of the prime emotions of darkness you can observe your thoughts, their energy, and where they lead, which will be unfolding into consequences which will be thoughts as well as bad feelings or unsettling memories.

With each emotion a corrupted thought will occur which will lead to a feeling of pain, as an emotion which caused the thought will therefore be a consequence which can be explained as a feeling. Hate will lead to a feeling of dislike, Fear will lead to a feeling of despair, Envy will lead to a feeling of insecurity, Lust will lead to a feeling of unfaithfulness and Anger will lead to a feeling of stress. Thoughts are feelings, just very difficult to sense sometimes. Memories, thoughts and emotions can be entwined or separate.

If any of these specks of darknesses are fully corrupted then it will lead to murder. While we can be under the influence of a corruption and stray from the path of perfection by indulging in emotions or consequences, which may lead to a minor crime the more the speck of darkness is magnified the greater the failing and the more corrupt you will be, therefore the resulting action will be intensified.

To be fully corrupted in all the negative emotions leads one to be truly evil and there is no spark of virtue in someone like that. The thoughts associated with these emotions are pain. There are different degrees of pain and it takes a keen observation to distinguish the subtleties associated with these inner spiritual meanings. Let me say that emotions like Lust gives rise to consequences that produce feelings that affect our memories. So, for instance if you have an emotion of Hate, this will lead to thoughts that cause dislike which will stir up feelings and memories which will come out in an action, though you may be totally unaware of what that action may be, for it may just be a certain gesture of the hand which will seem totally insignificant to you except if you are clairsentient and can sense energy then you will notice that this action is loaded with negativity. Then, and depending on how corrupted you become will lead to even more acts of evil.

Negative emotions, their thoughts, feelings and memories are painful even if your mind is so dull that you do not recognize this disturbance." The master stopped there to let his pupils try and comprehend what he had just warned them of. "Now, let us think of something more positive like the Virtue Manifest. The divine and holy sparks of light are our best chance of supreme perfection. These begin with, Love, Joy, Happiness, Hope and Goodness. All these are emotions and are sensations, as you should know by now they stimulate thoughts. The result is that Joy brings charity, Hope brings productivity, Happiness brings security, Love brings unity and Goodness brings kindness. All these results, of the primal emotive response to thoughts stir feelings and bring memories. So, if one experiences the emotion of Happiness which leads to a thought of security then a pleasant memory arises. This is a feeling of pleasure and the more you enhance the primal emotion the closer you are to perfecting it.

Once a virtue is perfected it destroys the speck of darkness related to the opposite of the virtue, for there is a balance. I will explain. The opposite of Anger is Joy. Then you have Love/Hate. Where Fear is the opposite of Hope. Happiness has an opposite called Envy, and finally Lust is the opposite to Goodness. A clear example would be to say that Anger breeds stress which is a negative feeling associated with memories and it is hard to be charitable when in this state. Hate breeds dislike and it is hard to maintain a relationship with this negative feeling, so therefore unity becomes difficult. Lust, breeds unfaithfulness and there is no kindness in infidelity. Fear, breeds despair and if you are in a state of anxiety it is hard to be productive. Finally, Envy leads to insecurity which is the complete opposite of happiness. This may be a lot to take in but you have your notes and I will hand out papers at the end. But, for now I will continue...

The emotions of corruption will grow more if you entertain evil, and the emotions of virtue will be enhanced if you exercise your will in the right way. None of us are born supremely perfect or completely corrupted, but we have a combination. This combination is the beginning of our destiny and is shaped by our environment, the way we are treated and our own internal choices, in other words we are given a chance, but it is not completely arbitrary. We have to nurture our virtuous emotions and control our negative ones which are the root of all our experiences.

If we can master a virtue then we will have defeated the Ultimate Corruptor on one principle. Meaning that if you perfect a virtue its opposite can no longer exist, so to perfect love, there will no longer be hate. Also, you can have love and hate co-existing together, but if you manifest the speck of darkness, negative emotion, to ultimate corruption then love will be destroyed and you will murder. But to sense discreet sensations we need to be aware of experiences and then to recognize actions which contain minute amounts of positive or negative energy.

There is a slight sadness to this uniqueness of human nature and that is that the struggle between the Ultimate Corruptor and the Virtue Manifest. People with two corrupting principles and two virtuous principles are said to have an equal balance of light and darkness, though their individual degrees may be out of harmony, they will be still said to be in a balance because the virtue has not been destroyed. If the spark of light, which is the source of virtue is destroyed it can be regained by an act contrary to the ultimate corruption, therefore planting a seed which will need nurturing and once more the force of the Ultimate Corruptor will be frustrated. Even a balance, though never perfect, for only virtue supreme is so, will be subject to the repercussions of their experiences, because of the varying degrees of unsettled conflict, and sadness is a universal mood that is blended around an uneven amount of either principle. If there is more corruption than virtue there is sadness. If there is more virtue than fault there is sadness.

I will explain. The more darkness there is the more the light is fading and sadness is also deepening into sorrow and misery. But, also if there is more virtue than corruption sadness will be present for the more light there is the keener it feels the pain of the unholy presence. Where there is much perfection there is also more responsibility therefore sadness is multiplied. This can drive someone into the depths of madness. Though, fragments they may be, such turbulence can cause one to experience the opposites more acutely.

There is a saying about sadness which I will share with you and it will comfort you if you can master it. *When one is alone in sadness it is suffering, but if one can be completely accepting of oneself, for the right reasons, then the loneliness becomes solitude.* This means that one has become happy with oneself in loneliness, so that the person will have gained all the virtuous principles, though there might still be corruption the power to hold the keys to life's turmoils where you will be able to see, with your eyes closed, all the stars in the darkness. Then, you will truly be the master of your own destiny.

So, therefore if you can achieve complete dissolution of all the negative emotions, meaning the corruptible darknesses and have complete virtue manifested then you will be truely perfected. The way to achieve this is to cultivate the sparks of light which are the positive emotions talked about. Joy, Happiness, Love, Hope and Goodness, not one of these are more important than the other, they are each priceless." Master Onis paused before saying, "Any questions? Please raise your hands."
Several of the pupils raised their hands in eager anticipation to ask the wise master some befuddling questions, but the master snapped back at them saying, "I am not answering any of your questions! If you would have listened properly and understood what I have said you wouldn't have any questions. I told you all absolutely everything you need to know! Now, there are copies of the lecture on this table, come and collect them... *all of you!* Even those who didn't raise their hands, you couldn't have taken it all in. There are decades worth of study here and I don't expect many of you to succeed. But.... there is hope." With that the master just strolled out of the room, with a concerned solitary smile at his performance, to the astonishment of everyone present.

The next morning the lord could be seen walking the grounds taking notes on where the dust from the *building of decay* was at its worst and getting the students to sign a petition on demolishing the building. He knew Faramel would be against it for in a recent conversation the imp had stressed the importance of the structure saying that the Lord of Death could only be comfortable surrounded by decay. But, the lord disagreed saying that it had become a burdensome part of his life and was beginning to feel uneasy with decay and morbidity. One student was a bit more fore coming than the rest and said, "Surely, you have the power to do whatever you want, for after all you are the Lord of Death and this castle?"

The lord then replied, "Just sign the petition and if beetles could dance then scotch would have no need of rashes."

"What do you mean?" the young man said.

"What I mean is that with the building gone slime won't hesitate to slip you up even if you are wearing socks."

The student frowned and wondered why he wasn't getting any sense out of the lord. He thought that this being the first time he had met him he was always like this. Faramel, then strolled up and said, "Lord, would you like to come with me to see if the *yomin* eggs have hatched. We are expecting two fluffy *yomin* lizards today."

"Well, imagine that! Two scrimping scurriers to go," and the lord followed Faramel only after he had the imp sign the petition.

When the sun in the sky was lowering, its brightness fading to set the sky off with pink clouds there was a knock on the door of Dorian and Nolon's room. Then, the imp Faramel opened it and walked in. Nolon, put down a book on 'The Warrior and the Deception' and Dorian looked up from cleaning *steelfang* the sword. "Greetings," the imp said in a warm manner.

"Hello," Dorian said and Nolon was expecting Dorian to go and see the Lord of Death, but Faramel then said, "I have a matter of urgent business. You are both called to the room of prophecy."

"What for?" enquired Nolon.

"You will be informed of this reason when you get there," the imp then said, "Follow me."

The boys then left their room and walked out of the building across a courtyard and on for another fifteen minutes until they came to a light sandy stoned building. Upon entering and following a little fairy with a ball of fire on a stick which lit the way they entered into the room of prophecy. Inside this room there were about twenty students all standing in a circle around the three masters. Dorian and Nolon joined the circle and waited. Eventually, master Shein spoke up, "It was a matter of urgency that you have all been called

49

here. We have discussed at length the seriousness of what we are asking you to do and it is at the utmost importance that you succeed in the request we ask of you, and of course you are free to decline the offer. A terrible thing is happening to our great Lord of Death who resides here at the *castle of fateful night*. Some of you may be aware of his behaviour and it is a cause for alarm for he has slipped into insanity and madness." There were some gasps of shock and muttering arose amongst the students. Master Shein then continued, "As now you understand the situation we have decided to send twenty one of our students to venture forth into the universe to recover jewels for the crown of death. Three of the jewels have been extinguished in the crown and each one represents a virtue or a corruption. There are ten jewels in all and one more which is the *universal gem of sadness* that is at the centre of the crown. Now, due to the nature of the *ceremony of fearsome divinity*, when the lord was changed from a human into the skeletal form of the Lord of Death, his virtues had been the source of his strength which has allowed him to stay in relative sanity for so long, though he had not completely eradicated all of his corruptions this was known to bring eventual instability. But, the ceremony continued for it was necessary and agreed upon. Now, we need to locate, in total, eleven jewels that are not found on this world. They are scattered throughout the universe and we have chosen twenty one of our students from all levels of competence and age to undertake the mission. We must succeed or when all the jewels are extinguished a sickening disease that is bound by their spell will emanate out of its confinement and scourge the land. The life of our lord is also at risk and he may never return from the depths of madness."

Master Onis then spoke, "So, we have chosen all of you to go on this quest. We will give you twelve days to contemplate and decide whether you want to undertake this mission, for it is no light choice and of course you will face dangers."

There arose a cacophony of voices as the masters left and Azul upon noticing Dorian and Nolon walked over and said, "Hi. What do you think of this business?"

Dorian said that it was a scary prospect but the opportunity to visit other worlds was fascinating and he wouldn't miss it for the world.

Nolon just summed it up in one word, "Awesome"

Coruja, the owl, who is the author of the prophecies, sat on a satin cushion reading a scroll with his glasses on. He was deep into his reading when there came a knock on the door. Within a few moments Faramel the imp entered and bowed down before him. "I have come to know if you have any revelations." The owl Coruja could not speak but held a pen in its claws and scribbled down some words. The imp took the paper and read it. *'The crown of death will be taken by an evil one who is not worthy of it.'* This gave Faramel a shadow of fear that passed over him, for who would steal the crown? He immediately thought that he would have to recruit some guards to keep watch over it. The owl then returned to reading the book and turned a page as the imp closed the door and headed out to see the masters to consult them on matters of great importance.

Zronisk, kept a calm composure as he unravelled the scroll of magic containing a spell of *screaming fire*. In front of him was his undead army of forty three specimens of a human nature and twelve undead dogs. A great bowl of unholy water lay in front of him and he recited the words on the parchment. The air vibrated with a crackling energy and a fire appeared swirling and descending into the unholy water. When the spell was complete the scroll disintegrated and the ashes fell into the dark water. The other followers of corruption watched on without the faintest hint of pleasure or satisfaction. Their dark leader, Zronisk motioned the others, by a wave of his hand, to give the undead the elixir now ready which will give the undead the power of magic, the force to execute *screaming fire* a spell that had immense consequences on living matter. One by one the dark ones sprinkled the unholy water on the undead army and a red fire hissed on them with serpentine flickers of flame crawling around their forms.

Zronisk, performed one last spell, the properties were to give this undead legion the power of semi rational thought. This meant that part of their brains will be made alive, no matter how rotten it had become, and this would give him the advantage of being more accurate with intructions. After the final necessary ingredient, Zronisk, stood in front of the tableau of horror and commanded in a voice used to giving orders, "We are going to attack the *castle of fateful night* and once we are there you are going to kill anyone who crosses your path. I have given you magic so you can destroy anything. Once, my mission is complete you will receive a thought, this thought will be, *return to the dark church*. When you hear this return here and wait." There was then a roar of undead appoval as the zombies understood their mission and had a passion to take life. A bat died of a heart attack and dropped from the ceiling and landed in the bowl of unholy water with a splash. Zronisk, looked at the floating corpse and then pulled it out. Then he muttered a few words and the bat came to life shivering with magic fire. "I will call you Morcego and you will be my eyes." Then he let the bat go and it flew out of a broken window towards the castle.

Master Onis aired his concerns, "I am not so sure that it is a wise thing that we send the three from the recently chosen to go to the other worlds. They have not completed their training and are unequipped to deal with what we might expect."
The master Quintok said, "Well, the prophecy demands it. Coruja, has never known to be wrong before and there must be a reason."
Shein, then spoke, "It will be dangerous, but they have the protection of the Virtuous Creator.
"Yes, but if anything should happen to them, well..." master Onis trailed off.
"We must trust," said master Shein. "There must be a reason."
The three then walked to the fencing arena to observe the students at sword play and master Quintok spoke saying, "I feel uneasy about this and I think I would feel better if we send someone along with Dorian, Nolon and Azul."
"Do you have anyone in mind?" asked master Onis.
"I was thinking of Slonic. He is skilled and can be their guardian."
"I agree," said master Onis. "It is far too dangerous for them alone."
Master Shein nodded and thought about the perils they might face and the dangers they might encounter, "Yes, it would be for the best."

Morcego, the bat, flew through the night and the magic from the unholy water hissed and crackled around him. The houses below were mostly in darkness and there were few people around and the bat glided effortlessly through the dark until the castle walls came in to view and Morcego flew up to one of the towers and looked around. Zronisk, could see the students walking the ground with lanterns and some were casting light spells; practising their magic. The bat flew around the grounds being the eyes of the corrupt follower.

The Lord of Death went for a walk and was mumbling to himself about anti clockwise and uncle jester. He had no idea that things weren't normal and was wearing the crown of upturned skulls on his head hearing the thoughts of others by its magical power. Making his way to the gardens he sat and watched two combatants practice their swordsmanship with wooden swords. When he tired of this he pulled out a small computer which he had purchased on another world and the screen lit up and a game called, *creepy crawlies* came on and he began to direct a spider into a cave, hopping over holes and swinging on thread across chasms. After about an hour he put the game away and climbed the steps onto the battlements and looked out across the vista. A sudden urge to run suddenly came over him so he jumped down over the wall and out of the castle and ran around the wall that secured the inhabitants of the great castle three time before finding a rope swing on a tree. Swinging for about half an hour on the rope which went over a deep ditch the crown flew off his head and got caught on a branch. This, didn't really concern the lord and some fireflies were zooming around so he thought about following them thinking that they would lead him to a secret rainbow where he could drink it and fly. But, there was no such rainbow and he eventually climbed the walls of the castle thinking that he was some sort of sneaky skeleton that would regain the sunlight before the hour was through, but, it was nearing midnight and there was no chance that the sun would rise just for him in half an hour.

Dorian awoke in the middle of the night when a great explosion reverberated through the walls. He then heard shouts outside and then Nolon arose also. They peered out of the window and could see fire burning. A section of the castle barracks was on fire and the bell began to toll. "That's the bell that signifies we're under attack," said Nolon. They both got dressed quickly and Dorian reached for *steelfang* and both of the boys ran out of the room and down the stairs; out into the night. In the courtyard there could be seen electric orange flames sprouting from the hands of the undead zombies as they sent blasts into the castle's defenders. Dorian, at first, stood terrified as an animated zombie lumbered towards him, then Nolon, used to wielding a weapon drove his sword into the undead monster, it fell to the ground and then got up again, no sign of any pain or blood. Dorian, then hacked an arm off with his magic sword and the zombie screamed an unholy curse as the magic of *steelfang* made it feel pain. The undead creature then let out a stream of unholy fire that caught them both and they fell to the ground in agony. As the zombie reached out to strangle Dorian, because he was the threat, Nolon sliced it with his sword and this gave Dorian time to thrust *steelfang* into the monster and it fell lifeless to the ground. "One down, and a horde more to go," Nolon said pointing to a small army of the undead battling the inhabitants of the *castle of fateful night*. A young zombie boy with a steel hand came up behind Dorian and clasped his fingers around his neck trying to crush his windpipe. Nolon, turned and struck out at the undead boy and the young zombie lad showed no sign of pain. A flow of magic escaped from the undead and Dorian screamed in pain; in a moment of fear he swung around and sliced the boy's face with his sword. The undead boy howled in an unimaginable and unholy shriek releasing his grip on Dorian. Nolon, sliced off his leg at the knee and the zombie boy went down unable to rise, so

53

they left him there and moved away from the ghastly pale face of the undead lad who had a rotting countenance which would stay in their memories for life. Slonic, then came up to them breathing heavily with a sword in one hand. "Looks like you've both managed to dispatch one of them," he said pointing to the lifeless corpse on the ground. "Yeah, it was a bit of trouble," Nolon said, and Dorian agreed. A lightning like thread of fire flashed past them and Slonic turned to see three of the undead approach. He ran towards them with Dorian and Nolon wielding weapons. One of the zombie's heads went flying as Slonic decapitated the rotting skull from its body and the head rolled then came to a halt and it started to let out a scream which didn't stop. Nolon, severed a hand before being struck down with a sickly orange fire. Dorian, pierced a heart which stopped the animated corpse and it collapsed to the ground, his magic sword draining its lifeforce. Slonic, was amazed at how easily they fell under Dorian's blade. After they had dispatched the three Slonic crushed the screaming head for it was still uttering an awful noise. "Take Nolon to the healing rooms, before he dies," Slonic commanded and Dorian picked up his friend who was unconscious and headed for the healing rooms. There was a clear path to the rooms of healing and Dorian had no encounters. Though, the screaming and noise of battle were all about. Master Quintok saw him as a zombie came from out of the dark, and cast an undead holy defensive spell around Dorian and the creature's hands went to Dorian's neck to strangle him from behind, the undead's hands dissolved at the touch. Master Quintok then realized that there were other zombies approaching and said to Dorian, "Be quick, get out of their sight." Dorian, hurried into the building and slammed the door closed behind him and laid Nolon down. There were no others here and it was dark, so he lit a candle and searched for healing herbs to ease Nolon's suffering for he was groaning and moving as if in a delirium. The door suddenly burst open and an undead monster groped his way through the dark and was about to summon a *screaming fire* spell when it collapsed in a fury of flames and screamed until it was completely made into ash. Azul, stood at the doorway. "Thanks," said Dorian. "Is he badly hurt?" she asked.
"I don't know, but he is still breathing," Dorian replied.

Zronisk and his dark followers, sent fireballs into some of the defenders burning and scorching them and the zombies continued their relentless attack. Master Quintok had animated the gargoyles from the chapel and they flew with stony swords and confronted the undead dogs that were tearing at the defenders in a crazed maniacal fury. The scene was one of destruction as some of the buildings had been set on fire to cause confusion and panic. The building of decay came in to view and the corrupt leader sent his undead monsters towards it, clearing a path for him to gain access. Two students versed in swordplay hacked and stabbed at the creatures until, caught off guard, one student dropped to the ground with his arm ripped from its socket; screaming in agony as he fell. The other scared for his life ran. Once inside the master of the undead teleported into the throne room where he expected to confront the Lord of Death, but he was not there and no matter how hard he searched he could not see or find the crown.

At this moment in time the Lord of Death was having a shower, using bubble bath to scrub his bony legs and skull, he was humming a tune called, soggy rat, and was completely oblivious to the commotion and war that was raging outside.

Defeated, Zronisk, gave the telepathic message, *return to the dark church*, to his zombie army. They retreated and Morcego the bat returned to the shoulder of the dark master as he walked to the east exit of the castle grounds. As his undead monsters lumbered on Zronisk, once out of the castle, noticed something hanging in the tree, it was the crown, 'How could that have got there,' he thought and reached up to take it. Now, a wave of satisfaction overcame him and he thought about putting the crown on but decided to wait until the time was right and he was at ease in his unholy church.

When the battle had died down and all that was left was the stinking corpses of the slain undead and the wounded students, master Onis ordered that the maimed and hurt be brought to the healing rooms. Inside, Dorian had no success in rousing Nolon and master Onis used a specific herb in conjunction with a liquid which soon awoke the dazed Nolon. "It's over," Dorian said. "They're gone."

"What did they want?" the young Nolon asked.

Master Onis replied saying, "They probably came for the *crown of death*. There was a prophecy."

Nolon, winced in pain and said, "Did they get it?"

"I don't know, but it is likely that the lord has kept it safe."

'There are seven dead from the castle inhabitants, which is unfortunate,' thought master Shein, 'But the undead were a count of thirty three. Though, the sickening horror of it all will remain in the minds of many, especially the young zombie lad who was a perversion of nature and morality.'

The wounded were cared for and healed. The dead were cremated and sent on the winds to inhabit dusty corners of *Skyworld* the planet. A putrid stench emanated from the undead corpses and they were soaked in a solution of petals from a plant to prepare them for burial. Dorian, was intrigued about the zombies and asked master Onis how it could be that they were reanimated. The master replied by saying, "There are various ways to bring back the dead into the world of the living. One of these ways are known by spell casters, but also there is another way. The blood of a crying statue can, with the use of a certain spell, bring back the dead."

Dorian, then remembered the statue of Ofelia in the church near his house and thought if they had used it to raise the dead and if so was it because Martiv didn't keep his mouth shut as he promised he would.

It was still early in the small hours when Dorian and Nolon finally got some sleep. Azul, in her room shivered, though she knew it wasn't the cold but the fact that they were assaulted by a horde of undead monsters. The window rattled in the breeze and chilled her thoughts before she finally fell into a restful slumber.

The Lord of Death was going through phases of rational thought, and delusional behaviour which would cause Faramel concern. While he was sitting in front of the high definition television the lord flicked through the channels to view the deaths of many. Usually he would be wearing the crown so he could read their thoughts and select an evil one to send Juiz the rat to go and judge. There was a particular individual who was pasty in complexion with greasy dark hair and a scar above his left eye; he was cursing and beating a child with a metal rod. The child screamed and bled until she didn't move any more. The lord saw that she was near death and grew angry with that nasty man. Jotting down the reference number which was XH34499. Faramel, then entered the room and the lord said, "Give this to Juiz and say he has black hair and a scar above his left eye and this man deserves it." The imp left the room and went in search of the rat. Juiz, was found in his quarters polishing a lens for his telescope and Faramel handed him the piece of paper with the destination reference number on it. "Another job?"

"Yes," replied the imp, "The lord said he deserves it."

"So far, the ones I have judged all deserve it.." the rat Juiz said.

"Well, it is a rather grim business," the imp said and then left the room.

Juiz, prepared a sandwich before donning his cloak and tapping his *mino* ring and saying the code XH34499. Instantly he appeared on another world in front of a small house with its door open. The rat pulled out a badge with the symbol of the *castle of fateful night* which was an owl reading a book and entered the house. It was dark inside even though it was mid afternoon. All the windows were closed and shutters kept the light out. A young girl lay on the floor curled up and was breathing softly. Juiz, noticed that she had many scars and fresh beating marks. A man sat on a chair and with his keen night vision Juiz could see that this was the man to be judged. He had damp black hair that stuck to his pale skin and a nasty scar above his left eye. He was awake and Juiz the rat sneaked around the shadows saying, "Preee...Ordainnnn..edddd." The man snapped out of his dreaming, "Who's there?.."

Juiz, crept closer, "Byyyy.."

"What do you want? If it is you Jannik I'll hit you..." the man started to get angry.

The rat drew even nearer, "Deathhh..." After this was said Juiz appeared in front of the man and flashed the symbol of the *castle of fateful night* at him. There was a flash from the badge and the man's eyes suddenly went blind and all he could see for a few moments was the sign of the owl reading a book, imprinted in the darkness of his sight. He gasped in shock and stood up bewildered and angered. He stumbled over the small stool that was in front of him and crashed to the floor. Juiz, left and another person was judged. The rat knew that the man's blindness would serve him right and it was a cruel punishment for a cruel person. His job was done the man was sightless for the rest of his life, and maybe he will learn a bit of humility thought Juiz.

There followed three days of mourning for the dead of the *castle of fateful night*. Prayers were said and there were readings in the chapel of the Virtuous Creator. Dorian, didn't know any of the slain personally but he felt sad because they were other students and he thought it could have easily been him that was cremated. The priest at the chapel had explained that the bodies of the slain were cremated because their ashes were blown on the wind to disperse, this was symbolic of the need to fly and explore the world. The zombies were buried because they were the dead of simple folk and not of the faith of the Virtuous Creator. Tradition had it that the soul would be freed from the mortal body through fire.

The Lord of Death was doing the washing up in the kitchen and was scrubbing a plate with a sponge. Dri, the elfling popped in and started a conversation with him. "So, what do you think of the attack on the castle?"

The lord replied, "Oh, it was a minor inconvenience. I was trying to have a peaceful shower when it kicked off and to tell you the truth a weasel is best taught how to jump then run around in circles."

Dri, didn't understand that and tried a new line of conversation, "So, why do you think they attacked? The gold in the treasury was not taken and nothing seems to be missing."

"Oh, they were probably bored or wanted a cockroach to keep them company," the lord sighed in sadness, "And, they were unclean," he said whilst cleaning a fork. "Which meant that they needed to dip themselves in the river for a complementary snack."

Dri, was baffled and reached for a cookie on a plate on the table. The lord turned and said, "Just one cookie per tooth, and don't blame me if they fall out."

"What? My teeth?" Dri said.

"No no. The chocolate in the cookies will fall out because they are dazed by the shiny teeth and are afraid of the belly."

Dri, smiled and walked away with a couple more of the biscuits leaving the lord to finish the dishes.

Dorian, under the tutelage of master Onis was preparing a solution that when mixed with plant material would become an effective healing balm. Master Onis gave particular attention to Dorian for he knew of the quest he had to undertake which would begin within the next couple of weeks. The master approached Dorian and said, "You have learnt quickly how to nullify poisons and heal wounds. Now, you must learn how to make potions that enable one to fly and others that give you the strength of ten men. These skills will complement you on your quest with Nolon and Azul."

Ceasing his work on stripping a plant of its leaves Dorian looked up at the master and stood up. "That sounds interesting," he said.

"Yes," the master replied. "It is a bit tricky sometimes to find the right plants to make these potions but you will be taking a selection of medicinal herbs and such with you on your journey. So, you should be well prepared." They walked to the back of the class where, on a table, a book was open on a particular page with pictures to instruct how to make a flying potion. Dorian, sat down there as the master gave guidelines as to make the elixer.

When the lesson had finished he headed to the fountain where he had planned to meet Azul and Nolon. There they talked of things of what they had been learning and Nolon who had a fresh cut on his arm let Dorian sprinkle some dried leaf on it and rub some lotion which immediately soothed and took away the pain, healing the skin and there was no sign of any hurt. Azul said, "Neat trick."

Nolon, then said, "I don't think that will be the last time Dorian heals my wounds if we go to other worlds where I have been reading that some of the beasts that live there are mightily ferocious.

They talked a little more until the bell of the chapel rang out and Dorian said that he was going to attend before supper. Azul, also showed her interest and accompanied Dorian there. Nolon, headed off to the library to research forging weapons and blacksmith's skills.

Inside the chapel of the Virtuous Creator there was a sweet scent of incense and Dorian placed the herb as being from a plant not grown on the castle grounds but he was familiar with it from his studies, it was called *nalder*. The two friends sat next to each other and were silent, taking in the atmosphere as others entered and took to their places.

The priest walked up to the dais and stepped up to welcome everyone for their yearning to know of the Virtuous Creator. There were small hymnals handed out and they all turned to a selected page and began to sing a praising tune called, All Our Love. Azul, seemed to know the melody and words for her hymnal remained closed and she didn't falter with the words. After three uplifting songs they all sat back down and waited as the priest announced that he would now talk of the corruptions evident in humankind; throughout the world:

HATE. A speck of darkness that corrupts can be the negative emotion of hate. It is devious and the unholy evil ones seek to magnify it so as to ultimately corrupt and destroy the virtuous spark of love. When you dislike someone or something, this comes from the darkness of hate. There are negative consequences of this because it interferes with our striving for unity. It is commanded of us to marry and raise a family but, hate is a strong emotion and seeks to undermine the virtue of love. Many an unhappy marriage has ended in separation because of the intense feelings of dislike which came from hate. Where love strives to bring together and it upholds the principle of everlasting unity, hate will destroy and bring ruin unless you are very careful. So, even though it is difficult to destroy the negative speck of darkness that is hate, beware of its influence and try not to dwell on it too much for that will enhance it. Even though there are successful marriages when this speck is present, do not let it rule or become stronger than the virtue of love otherwise things will go wrong for you.

FEAR. The negative speck of darkness known as fear is despairing. One knows that this is counter productive meaning that it is difficult to succeed or achieve much when one is fearful. This can get in the way of being able to feel good and disarms all hopes of advancement in life. But, cultivate hope with the exercise of faith so that you have dreams that you want the opportunity to become of fruition. Beware of your thoughts because fearing is tricky to identify and will lead you to despair threatening your plans and causing doubt to multiply.

ENVY. The speck of darkness called envy is a subtle energy. It works its way into our experiences and leads us to feel insecure and when there is happiness, envy has no place. When you feel envy it can lead you down paths that you shouldn't be walking. It arises in one, bad emotions and these are painful whether you recognize the pain or not. When one is envious one wants to be better or achieve more, this is not good because one is insecure and will need to prove or get what one is envious for. Learn to be happy and envy will depart. Be grateful for the small things in life and learn to respect and be joyful of another's success, for envy has been the insecurity of many and can affect our life in more ways than one, so cast it out and have no more to do with this darkness.

LUST. The darkness of lust brings infidelity. One cannot live life with this speck of darkness and be completely kind. For, even if you are just unfaithful to one person, there is great pain. Sometimes, pain is not recognized because emotions are hard to evaluate. If one is unfaithful when the darkness has become apparent, whether it be of a relationship or a gain that you may want, it diminishes your kindness and has established corruption. Your voice will become affected with unkindness even if you show kindness to one person, another will be the receiver of a cruel tongue for lust is ever wanting and will want what you think you need. Be careful then to examine your intentions for gain because they may be tainted.

ANGER. The negative aspect of anger will be stressful when this darkness is present. When someone is angry it is difficult to be charitable to another and will be more onerous to give, this is not good because it will affect your judgement, so don't justify your anger because it seems righteous. It is a thing of no worth and can only bring negative consequences. To live with anger is an undesirable thing because it will corrupt your charity so that what you give is not of much worth, but give anyway as your virtue becomes more. Your anger is weighed with every charitable act and with some the more given is less than the meagre offering of a poor man. Do not be angry then when you give and when the reaction is one that does not please you, for your joy will increase when you least expect it and all is not what it seems and your reward you will not recognize as the act in which it was given for.

When his speech was over it left them all thinking of how best to live with the knowledge that corruption is a real negative part of everyday life. The priest's final words were that to be aware of these things is the first step in being able to combat them. Then, a final hymn was sung called, A Loving Father. Azul, walked out with Dorian and they made their way to the great hall to have supper. Talking all the way there Dorian was interested to know that Azul was brought up in a religious family and that she had the most respect for the majestic Holy Father who is the Virtuous Creator.

Zronisk, had the *crown of death* on his head and was listening to a cacophony of sounds which were the thoughts of every living being. Alien sounds and languages filled his mind and he took off the crown after a few minutes of unbearable noise. He thought to himself that there must be a way of separating the babble to hear a coherent thought of an individual. But, the technique he thought must be straight forward, for the Lord of Death, as Zronisk knew, usually had an empty mind, maybe that was the key he thought, so placing the crown aside and thinking of trying later after his head ache had gone he went to get a book of meditation which was stolen from a monk who was a stranger in the land. Morcego, the bat sat perched by a window peering out and observing two men and a little dog walking along the road past the unholy church.

On this day Dorian was instructed to get *steelfang* the sword and Azul and Nolon were also called from their classes to the fencing arena where master Quintok was awaiting them. "Now, you know that there will be great peril on your travels into other worlds.. So, I have called you here to train you in what little time we have left. I will use magic that can take form so Nolon when you hit a creature you will feel your blade make contact. I do this so that you will not be caught off guard with real combatants." Instructing them to stand close to each other and giving Azul a weapon he said, "Now, fear is your enemy so remain calm and try your best." A moment passed before master Quintok summoned a horde of grotesque alien creatures with claws and venomous stings. In an onrush of adrenaline the three young pupils braced themselves as the horde charged them. Nolon, was quick and ran at them swinging his sword cutting deep into the alien and swinging his shield around to block a clawed hand. Dorian, stood there in fear and couldn't move, until Azul nudged him and three of the alien hybrids were almost upon him until he swung his sword around to slice one. Azul, tried to use the weapon but found it clumsy and the alien bit into her leg, she didn't feel any pain and stuck her sword into it and the creature dropped down lifeless. Then, she threw a ball of acid at the others and they screamed in unison before dissolving in a bubbling mess on the floor. Master Quintok, applauded. "Well, done. Your magic has saved you. Dorian, you need to work on your reaction time and

Nolon you are a bit of a loose cannon but your bravery is exceptional." They spent the next two hours going over scenarios that tested their abilities and Azul learnt how to hold the sword correctly, so as to use it more efficiently.

After the exercises were over their minds were buzzing with strategies and battle formations which were used to eliminate any possibility of advantages that their enemies could have against them. Nolon, saw the reasons behind this and was convinced that master Quintok knew what he was teaching them, although his usual tutor, master Shein, held more respect for him because he knew everything that there was to know concerning warcraft, but Azul said, "Master Quintok has an uncanny ability to know weaknesses in us and I am sure that this is important for our survival."

Dorian, agreed and said, "Yes, it is mentioned somewhere in the book of Everlasting Truths that to know our weaknesses is a strength which with thought we can become wiser. I think that it says that no one is without fault but to know your failings allows us to turn them to our advantage and succeed in life."

Nolon, who hadn't read much of the holy book looked pensive and said, "I agree. There was a book that I was reading of great heroes in battle and a man, who I forget his name, didn't focus on his short comings and it was the death of him. We are taught things that improve our skills so we don't have any weak techniques or defensive manoeuvres. One particular teaching to have a good balance is to know how to be off balance so that it improves our composure. There is some truth in that holy book and it is, I have noticed, been echoed in our instructions."

Dorian, nodded and as the three of them walked toward the main entrance of the great hall, tired and hungry the bell rang for the students to gather there for their evening meal.

The days passed quickly and anticipation grew steadily as the time approached for the three to travel through space and to new worlds. Upon the evening before their departure the three masters addressed the students and master Onis spoke saying, "Tomorrow, will bring you to the first step of your journeyings. I will say that it will be dangerous for some and that there may be fatalities, so that some of you may not return. But, remember this, it is of utmost importance that you all are undertaking this adventure. As you know if the jewels in the crown of death are extinguished than a nasty insidious disease will be unleased on our world which could be the demise of us all. The lord is slowly losing his sanity and without him in his right mind he cannot attend the council of Mortis Divinus, which he will need to be at if there is going to be anyone to represent our galaxy for virtuous reincarnations. What this means is that there might be a shift in balance if he does not represent us and that the worlds around us and ours may become subject to a mass of evil incarnations bringing with it sorrow and pain to all virtue manifestations."

Some of the students already knew of this but for Dorian, Azul and Nolon, it was a matter that was not mentioned to them, and which left them thinking that it is important that they succeed and are quick about it. The master then went on to explain to each group of three that the jewels that need to be recovered are rare and difficult to find, but there had been some forethought and each group was given information that is written on a scroll to aid them in their search. Slonic, approached them and held out his hand in greeting, shaking each one in turn, then addressing Dorian he said, "I will be accompanying you in your travels." They all felt relieved that he was going to be with them and he pulled out a small metal box and handed it to Dorian saying, "If you slide the name plate which says, Everlasting Truths, then it will operate. By saying a word it will iterate the relevant passages in the holy book to you."

"Cool," said Azul, and Nolon looked awed.

"It is a gift from Coruja the author of the prophecies," Slonic said, "And, it should be of some use."

"Who?" asked Dorian.

"Don't you know of the owl Coruja?" Azul exclaimed astonished.

"No, I don't," Dorian replied crestfallen.

"Well," said Nolon, "You should!"

Slonic, then smiled and said, "He has probably been studying too much. Coruja is the *author of the prophecies* and every so often he presents a foretelling to the castle's inhabitants when it is necessary."

"Well, he hasn't done so since I have been here," Dorian said as if he were missing a special event that no one had told him about.

"There will come a time," was Slonic's response.

Azul, smiled and her eyes sparkled with amusement, "Don't worry he is said to have a life span of thousands of years so we can wait. Apparently, he reveals a prophecy at least once a year."

Dorian, felt better and Nolon suggested that they all go and prepare for the next day.

When in his room Dorian pulled out the small metal box that Slonic had given him and slid the name plate. Instantly, it opened and a stone owl was revealed wearing glasses with an open book on a lectern in front of it. Dorian then said, "Anxiety," for he was apprehensive of his travels the next day. Immediately, the pages of the small stone book turned and the owl spoke saying, "Anxiety is born of fear. Take away your thoughts on this worry and imagine a light in your heart. Remember your successes and turn your thoughts to all that you have achieved. Believe that you are being watched over and do not fear death for it comes upon us all at a time we cannot tell. So, do not fear but think on what you hope for. This, is worth the risk that brings fear. Uncertainty, will make you stronger when you are successful, so have hope for it is what helps us struggle through times of adversity." Dorian, switched the name plate and the metal box with the stone owl closed up. He paused to think on what had been said and felt better when a light shone in his heart for just a few moments there was peace and joy. Then his thoughts went to his hopes and there was fear there. Fear of not succeeding and failure. But, hope was there none the less and that gave him a spark of happiness, to know that his dreams were worth striving for. His hope lay on stopping the disease from the *crown of death*, also Azul crossed his mind. He found her naturally beautiful and felt a longing to hold her hand or see her blue eyes sparkle.

A morning sky greeted Dorian as he pulled open the curtains of his room. Nolon, was already awake and packed ready to go. "So, you are all ready then?" Dorian said noticing the pack on Nolon's bed. "Yes, I have a check list and I do believe I haven't forgotten anything," Nolon seemed content without a hint of discontent from the apprehensive journey they were going to begin this day. "Well, we have some time yet. It is not till after lunch that we leave our home planet Skyworld for the distant Turgon," Dorian said, and added, "It is going to be dangerous."
"Have no fear Dorian. We have the skills. The amount of extra studying we've done this past week or so should aid us in our adventures."
"Yes," Dorian said still feeling every doubt niggling him.
Nolon, left for breakfast as Dorian began to pack his stuff. He had also written a list and it didn't take long for him to gather his essential belongings, things that he thought he would need, like his clothes and some books, also he had all the herbs in his pouch which were mostly fresh; some small vials of liquid were there which would allow him to make certain concoctions. Noticing the small book on gargoyles which he had picked up on the way to the *castle of fateful night* he slipped it in his bag. After strapping *steelfang*, his magic sword in a scabbard around his waist he left for the great hall. On arriving Azul was there smiling sitting next to Nolon, then Slonic approached with his plate of fried food and sat down next to them. "You are all required at the room of Immortal Heroes precisely after lunch for our journey to Turgon. It will only take a few moments for us to travel there, so don't worry about that." Slonic, drank some milk with honey and mentioned that they

were after one jewel in particular. "The *crimson fire gem* is most precious and is only found on Turgon. The inhabitants there live most simple lives but in some parts of the world there is technology."

Nolon, spoke up saying, "Yes, and their language is difficult. Mainly a pictorial way of writing and to say hello is pronounced, *Yoni*."

They had all been introduced to the ways of this world and the customs, "But," Slonic pointed out, "Do not say it quickly, it is considered rude to be hasty in greetings."

Azul, then added, "But, it is okay to shake hands with the locals in the city of Rumin, though some of the tribes that live in the forests and deserts are offended if you touch them without asking them first and apparently can get quite nasty if one does so."

Dorian, also contributed to the display of knowledge by saying, "The flowering plant known as Henlese, which can be used as a substitute for eating, can be found in some of the forests, especially in the Uri woodlands. It can be used for up to two weeks without any other source of nutrition except water. Recognised by its velvety leaves and strong scent, with diamond shaped flowers."

"Well," Slonic said looking impressed, "I think you all know your stuff. It should be a simple mission and I expect we will return within the week."

The three spent the morning roaming the grounds of the castle and talking among themselves. A three eyed *mocos* bird flew down near them and observed their mannerisms before Azul noticed it and pointed out that it was a portentous omen to see one. "They are very rare and always foretell bad luck," she said.

Nolon, who was not a great enthusiast when it came to folk lore pointed out that there is a high possibility that we would see them some time here for they only live in this part of the world, very rarely do they travel any further."

Though Nolon was just pointing out a fact, Azul couldn't help but feel a shiver run down her spine and Dorian was somewhat uncomfortable with this sign. Eventually the bird flew off with its characteristic squawk as it rose into the air.

Zronisk, the corrupt, had the *crown of death* on his head. The previous attempt to keep his mind blank had ended in failure and the resulting headache was so severe that he hadn't tried to wear the crown for a little while. Once again he was forced to listen to a pandemonium of noise as a whole variety of language and speech filled his mind. Quickly he took off the crown before he ended up with a two day throbbing head as what had happened before. The relief was immediate and he tossed the crown onto the ground with unsatisfactory discontent. A thought occurred to him. He had an old friend. A goblin, who studied magical artefacts and was known to serve the Ultimate Corruptor. So, he wrote on a piece of parchment a short note for Groni the goblin to visit the unholy church and thereby view, and possibly assist Zronisk in using the crown for world dominating purposes. Tying the note to the bat's leg he let Morcego ready himself to flap his way to find the goblin Groni, the dark master gave thought impressions to the bat so it would find the way. Morcego, flew out of the broken window with the note and hastened towards its destination.

They were standing in expectation within a circle of light in the room of Immortal Heroes. The masters were observing; Dorian, Azul, Nolon and Slonic were bathed in a radiant glow as they were transported to the world of Turgon to search for the *crimson fire gem*. They were advised to keep their eyes closed for the journey, but Nolon was most curious and kept his eyes open, when he felt a warm breeze scented with wild flowers his vision took a while to adjust as he had been temporarily blinded by the travel glare. Azul, was the first to speak, "I am standing in a rainbow!"
Slonic, smiled and said, "Yes, it seems you are."
Looking around him Dorian took in the surrounding vista. There were unusual trees and an insect, the size of an apple, with tiny wings bumped into him and chewed his jumper before being yanked off and thrown into a bush.
They all wore a band of silver around their heads which was a *universal translator*, it could turn their speech to the local dialect and also received unusual languages in the common tongue of Skyworld their home planet.
Slonic, suggested that they head for the nearest city which was about three miles away over the nearest hills. He had studied some maps before his journey here and was a little familiar with the lands.
There was a little sun, but the cloudy sky burst forth sprays of rain every now and again. A stretch of trees to their right swayed as a gust of wind blew momentarily and Azul wrapped her cloak tighter around herself and said, "Are we expecting to get the jewel from the city we're going to?"
Slonic, seemed assured that it was a simple task and replied saying, "There should be an establishment selling rare gems and precious stones in the city. Most major inhabited areas will have tradesmen selling expensive metals and jewels. We should be back at the *castle of fateful night* by tomorrow evening if all goes well."
Nolon, resting his hand on the pommel of his sword said, "Will we be expecting any trouble?"

"No. It should be quite straight forward," Slonic assured him.

Then Dorian pointed to a lumbering hulk that was strolling down the hill in front of them about ten minutes walk away, "What is that?" he said.

Slonic, froze and exclaimed in a harsh breath, "It is a troll."

The creature had an axe slung over its shoulder and hadn't seemed to of noticed them. "What shall we do?" asked Azul.

"There is nowhere to hide," he said. "Let's hope it doesn't want any trouble."

"But.." started Nolon, "They are known for violence and destruction."

Slonic, nodded and said, "Yes, but they can sometimes be reasoned with."

The four travellers steered a little way around so that they wouldn't be directly in line with its path, but the troll looked up and headed toward them. "It has seen us," remarked Azul, a clear tone of worry in her voice. They halted and the green skinned troll held the axe in his hand and grunted a few words that were translated as, "Giv' us yore money!"

Slonic, stood up to him and said, "We have no money for you but there are some wild *gnoz's* in the woods over there," he pointed to the woodlands, "And they are tasty roasted," he said this to appeal to the troll's appetite, but instead it raised the axe and said, "Den U die!" It swung its axe at Slonic's head but went wide as he side stepped.

"So much for reasoning," Nolon said and drew his sword alongside Dorian. The troll swung his axe a few times before Slonic pierced his thick skin with a few inches of steel and Nolon hacked its hand off. Azul, then blasted it with a spell which made it explode everywhere. The mess was disgusting and Dorian said, "You over done it a bit there Azul."

"Yeah, it was about to die by my sword," Nolon said slightly disappointed.

"The main thing is we are out of trouble," Slonic, wiped the flat of his short sword on the troll's garments to get rid of the slimy blood.

"Shall we search it?" Nolon said.

"You can if you want, but I doubt if you'll find anything of worth," said Slonic shaking his head.

Nolon, stuck a hand in one of its pockets and pulled out a dead mouse. "That's gross!" Azul said wincing her face.

"It was probably a snack," said Slonic.

Nolon, looked to another pocket and saw a head of a lizard poking out drenched in a gooey liquid. "I don't think I'll bother searching it anymore."

They went on their way, leaving the dead troll where it lay.

It was a dark night when there came a knock on the door of the unholy church. A mute follower of corruption opened the creaky door and there stood the goblin called Groni. This goblin had travelled far and was specialized in magical artefacts. The hooded mute beckoned the untidy goblin inside and closed the door behind him. He led Groni into the main worship area where there was a small army of zombies seated upon rows of wooden benches, an eye of one fell out of its socket and a rat scurried away with it. Zronisk, was giving a sermon and made his point clear that.. "Suffering, is good for people and it is a joy to give someone pain, because everyone, people just deserve to suffer. So, it is our mission to cause as much mayhem as possible and yes, put as many miserable lives to death as one has energy for. Especially, the so called virtuous ones. They deserve to suffer the most. And, I'll tell you why.. They think that they are better than us and frankly they just need to be put in their place, a broken arm, nose or leg is supposed to work wonders on these sorts of people, though the stronger ones will still sing hymns and pray whilst you execute them, but remember this, out great unholy god is the source of all power and he has promised to give such power to the ones who follow him so we may bring others in to obedience to him..." Zronisk, paused as the congregation just decayed; a rotting hand fell off one; a few dribbled and Groni was the only one to give the dark master a round of applause as he stood up and walked towards the follower of corruption. "A fine speech," the goblin said, "And, the unholy one is most proud of you. I can tell by the way he has blessed the congregation. "Groni, you excel in mischievousness and may the unholy God give you strength to slay." They shook hands and Zronisk led him to the chamber of evil contemplation where there was a painting of an execution. They both sat down and Zronisk poured them both a drink of fizzy orange which was purchased from another world. "So," said Groni as he sipped his drink, "What's this I've heard about you having the crown of Death?"

"Oh," said Zronisk, "I acquired it of late but I can't seem to get it working." He rose and walked over to a skeleton that was propped up by some stones and removed the crown from its skull. "Here it is," he said handing it to the goblin. "It has some lights glowing but when I put it on all I hear is a cacophony of noise and I can't seem to read anyone's mind with it." Groni, took the crown and examined it. Then, he placed it on his head and immediately removed it. "Yes, I see your problem." The goblin turned the crown around in his hands scrutinizing it carefully, "There seems to be some lights extinguished in some of these jewels. This may be the source of your problem."

Zronisk, picked up his drink and had a mouthful of fizziness, "So what do I do? Is there any way to fix it?"

Groni, spoke in an even tone, "Well, it seems to me that you need to get some new gems. I did some research before I came down and apparently the jewels are symbolic of the five virtues and the five corruptions, according to the followers of the Virtuous Creator. Also, there is the jewel of universal sadness, which is also not shining, so there are five gems that need to be replaced." Morcego, the bat came fluttering down to the table and Zronisk impulsively picked it up and stroked it. "And, where would I find such precious jewels?" the dark master asked.

"I am not sure, but I could inquire into this and send a message via my winged arachnid to you," the goblin reached for his glass.

"You have a flying spider?" Zronisk said in admiration.

"Yes, I have experimented on creatures and altered their growing habits to produce things like a goat with three heads, a snake with a scorpion's tail, and a winged spider amongst other amusements," the goblin Groni held a hint of pride at this information and pulled out a centipede with the head of a fish, "This, may look harmless, but its teeth are venomous and the poison is fatal if it entered into a living body." The mutated fish thing went to bite Groni's fingers and he squeezed it to control it and the creature let out a small but audible whimper. Wrapping the monstrosity in a piece of reinforced cloth he returned it to his pocket. "But, what I find more interesting is power..."

Zronisk, nodded in agreement for they both were eager to dominate and control. "Yes," the dark master said, "Once the crown is working I will be able to impose my will more effectively. No one will be safe, even their inner most thoughts will be known. This will allow me to select the most loyal followers for world domination, and once I have this planet under my rule then I will enslave other worlds."

Groni, smiled at the sheer darkness of the undertaking his friend Zronisk was planning, "And, don't forget, the most unholy dark one will be most pleased with you and may even grant you immortality."

"Yes, I was hoping that," the dark master said, "For to conquer the galaxies.. it will take a while, but, my service to the great dark one has its rewards..."

The two chatted about torture and executions for another hour before Groni went on his way promising to send his pet, *creepwing*, to deliver a note when there is more known. Once the goblin had left the dark master sent Morcego to flutter off to the *castle of fateful night* to see and hear anything that may be of any use. He hoped that he could find out something about the crown and wondered if there was a search for it taking place.

It was nearing night as the adventurers reached the crest of the hill they were walking. They stopped for a few moments to regain their breath. Just below them, a city sprawled out with various lit dwellings. "Let us say a prayer," suggested Slonic, "We may need our Creator's guidance."

They all closed their eyes and Slonic began, "Our Virtuous Creator, may you be with us as we go into the city below. We ask you to continue to bless us with your love and we send you our love from our hearts so that you know it is our will to love you."

Then Nolon continued the prayer, "And Holy Creator, please make my sword swift if ever I need to use it."

Azul, added, "May you help us find what we are looking for so that we may return to Skyworld safely."

Dorian, then finished the prayer, "And, Holy One, as you know our thoughts and desires may you teach us your ways so that we may read the signs you send and to guide us in life, may your presence be known and your will be done."

They opened their eyes and unclasped their hands. Each had felt a warm loving spirit within them as the prayer came to a close and Slonic smiled saying, "Let us go down to the city and find somewhere to sleep." Azul, was humming a hymn and the four descended the hill along a path that had been worn by many feet. It was much easier to walk down hill and within the hour they were within the great city and people were wandering about. The four travellers took in the strange architecture and the unusual clothes the inhabitants were wearing. Slonic, saw a sign hanging over a tall house and stopped saying, "This might be a good place to stay." They went within the building and inside, in the front room there were several chairs and a couch. Nolon, sat down on the couch and Slonic, rang a small bell. A crooked man came from out the back and placed his hands on the counter, "Yes, can I help?"

"We are looking for a room for the night. How much do you charge?" Slonic, expected a twinkling in the man's eyes as if strangers would be taken advantage of and he would be calculating a higher than usual price, but the man was slow in speaking and said that it would be six bronze coins each for the night and that it would include supper which will be served in half an hour. So, Slonic paid the man in bronze and he showed them a room with five beds; a window over looked the road outside where trees were lined down it and birds were congregating in an excited manner. They left some of their belongings in the room before going down to the main dining area but Nolon refused to part with his sword, saying that he never knew when he would need it and that he wouldn't feel safe without it. In the main eating area there were several people at tables and a few at the bar. A small, dark green, warty creature with a long pointy nose was drinking a glass of milk. "What is that?" Nolon said to Slonic. He replied saying, "It is a goblin."

"What is a goblin doing here?" Nolon said disgusted.

"Well, they are welcome in some parts of this world," Slonic said smiling.

Dorian and Azul eyed the creature and when it turned to look at them they quickly averted their eyes. "Strange," said Azul and Dorian agreed. When food was brought to their table a man and a woman dressed in red went up to a platform with the goblin and they introduced themselves as Homn, Graiora and the goblinoid was called Flork. The two humans had instruments which they immediately started to pluck strings creating an interesting sound and the goblin began to sing. "Quite a good voice actually," Nolon said. Dorian, was impressed by the goblin and Azul was humming along. The words mentioned an ogre who had a broken heart and ended up marrying a goblin who was a princess. Slonic, let out a laugh every now and again hoping that he wouldn't offend Flork, for the singer looked most tearful as he sang.

When the performance was over a young boy and girl went around with a collection bowl and the diners gave money for the musicians. It was getting late by the time Nolon had ran out of things to say and tiredness crept into his speech. Dorian, yawned and Azul's eyelids were heavy. "Time to get some sleep," Slonic said, "And, in the morning our search will continue for the *crimson fire gem*." They made their way up the stairs and after unlocking the door they entered their room which had a scent of damp, so Slonic opened the window to let in some fresh air. The amount of walking they did eased their drift into dream land and within moments of getting into bed they were all sound asleep. In the dark of the night a strange sound came from the street below, followed by a scream. Dorian awoke and got up to see what could be the source of the noise. Looking out he saw a strange scene, there was a man on fire running, and being chased by what seemed like pack of dogs. He watched for several minutes before closing the window and slipping back into bed. It took a while before he fell asleep as he wondered who the burning man was and why he was being chased.

In the morning Azul was the first to awake and she got dressed and went for a walk to the square just down the road where it could be seen from the window. As she walked down the street there were traders with their shops open and people walking by. No one really took any notice of her though she thought her wand tucked into her belt might give some cause for concern, if they knew that she practiced magic. Sitting down on one of the wooden benches she observed the town's folk and watched a mouse slip into the side of a building where a sign hung saying, 'Bringot's Bakery." The mouse then reappeared with a thick crust in its mouth and scurried down the road and into another hole. A man passed with green shades of clothing, he carried a pad of paper and sat at the bench next to her and began to earnestly sketch away, drawing lines with a pencil. He looked up at Azul and said, "Have you seen anything interesting this morning?"

Azul, said, "Only a mouse."

The man smiled and replied saying, "Yes, it was probably Horase. He goes to the bakery every morning and gets his daily bread."

Azul, smiled also and wondered if anything in this town actually goes unnoticed, which led her to think that this artist is a very observant man. She sat for a while not really interested in making conversation until she decided to look at what the young man was drawing before leaving. "That's really good," she said in honesty, for the representation of the buildings was accurate. The man had started to draw in a dragon lying on the roof of the blacksmith's. "Just thought I would add something a bit out of the ordinary to this piece," he said with a slight hint of playfulness in his tone. Azul, then left the man to his work and returned to the house where Dorian was sipping honey and cinnamon milk at a table in the dining room. Slonic, walked in carrying a pamphlet and sat down next to Nolon. "So where did you wander off to this morning?" he said to Azul.

"Oh, I just went for a walk and sat in the square down the road to think," she said innocently.

"Well, I sensed that you were in no danger, but I think it is best if you let us know when you decide to disappear again," Slonic's tone was soft yet it held a quality of authority that she dared not to defy.

"Okay," Azul looked away and a serving maid brought her some toast and a cherry pie. Nolon, was looking at a procession of ants that had been marching along the side of the wall, which led toward the kitchen area. He felt that the ants were hungry so when he saw that no one was looking he threw a sugar cube over to them for he had heard that they liked sweet things, but the ants ignored the offering and continued their inexorable pilgrimage to where there was fresh food to be had. Nolon, a little disappointed picked up the leaflet that Slonic had placed on the table and read through some of it. Dorian, asked, "What's in that?"

Nolon's reply, after reading some of it, was, "Just some local news. Apparently there is a new shop opening on Hallmark Street, it is going to be selling fresh fish and vegetables. And, there is also a report of a murder which happened three days ago on the west side where a man was found beaten to death and the investigation continues." He put the booklet down and Dorian then read some of it. Slonic, was sitting out the front taking shavings off of a piece of wood that he was shaping into a dove in flight, waiting for the young ones to finish breakfast.

Morcego, the bat, found a place to hang upside down in a room where there were rows of chairs and a small table which served as a desk. Master Quintok was sitting on one of the chairs with a young student explaining to him about the uses of magic. Morcego, listened in for about half an hour until Zronisk got bored with the master and signalled to the bat to find someone else to eavesdrop on. So, Morcego flew out of the room and located another master who was in the midst of a group of students showing them how to defend oneself with a spear in close combat. He flew on until passing three young neophytes involved with a conversation about the *crown of death*. The bat hung from the tree above them and Zronisk listened as the trio talked. "Apparently, the jewels in the crown represent the virtues and corruptions."
"Yes, and then there is the *jade fire gem of universal sadness* which is the most precious, because all living things suffer and it is the key jewel that allows the lord to link into other people's minds."
A girl with pink tips on her hair added, "That's why the lord is losing it, because, you know, he has held the position of lord for many thousands of years and the gems are losing their power."
The boy with red cheeks then said, "And, I heard that he will be replaced." There was a moment of silence as the three took in this prospect."
"It would be so cool to be the Lord of Death. Imagine being immortal!"
They all agreed on the position that the Lord of Death held was prestigious and many would like to have the powers he had. The boy then said, "I wonder when Azul will be back from Turgon?"
"They are due back within seven days," the girl said, "Apparently Dorian is with them and he has a magical sword."
"How do you know that?" the other girl with a pony tail said.
"Well, Nolon told me. He beat my brother in combat and they got talking afterwards. Nolon said that magic weapons are really rare and that Dorian had a sword which had been embued with arcane properties."
"I think they will be safe," the boy said, "They all have abilities and the Virtuous Creator on their side."
"Yes, but the *crimson fire gem* is supposed to be a difficult jewel to find because it isn't formed naturally on that planet, but is supposed

73

to have been transported there by a meteorite from space many years ago."

"So, which quality does it represent?" the girl with the pony tail said whilst reaching for an apple from her bag.

The young girl with the pink tips on her hair closed her eyes momentarily, "I think it is the virtue of *hope*."

"And the others who went off are searching for the jewels of *hate, love* and *joy*," the girl with the pony tail said and then took a bite of the apple. The boy thought of the other worlds that the chosen few were on searching for the gems and felt a bit envious that he was not among them for despite the danger it was an opportunity for an adventure.

Morcego, flew away then, back towards the unholy church. Zronisk, knew all he needed to know and his mind was burning with the anticipation of acquiring the *crimson fire gem* for himself and that the prospect of gaining a magical sword in the process was also a thought that he relished.

The Lord of Death was on another world and he slipped his credit card into the cash machine and put in his security number. After three attempts the machine didn't accept the number and swallowed his card. So, he went into his bank and joined the queue, waiting to make a complaint, for he needed some cash to buy a present for Faramel the imp because it was his birthday soon.

It was late morning when Slonic and the other three entered the jewellers to enquire about the *crimson fire gem*. "Good day," came the greeting from the shop owner who was a little plump and sported a moustache. "How can I help?" he asked.

Slonic, put his request forward and the man immediately shook his head and said, "Sorry, but those gems are very rare and are usually found on the other continent, Ursulia. But, I can order one for you though it might take a few weeks and payment is of course, in advance."

"Okay," Slonic replied, "We will think about it and return if there leaves us no other option. Thank you for your time." The man then picked up a pen and continued to fill out a crossword that he was puzzling over as they left the shop. Azul, was admiring the rings in the shop window and Slonic said, "I don't think waiting for two or more weeks is worth our while we might be able to find the gem before then if we can get to Ursulia." As he finished his sentence a great hushing sound came from their left and turning, Dorian saw a space craft settle softly blowing up clouds of dust. Nolon, was awed at the sight for even though he had seen illusions of these space

faring vessels, now it was made real with the metallic sheen
reflecting the sun on its smooth surface. "It is a little unusual for this
part of the world," Slonic said referring to the fact that the main
space ports are on the other side of the world. "There is not much
trade here. I wonder what these folk want?" A door slid open and
two humanoids came out dressed in what looked like fine silk. They
had green eyes and surveyed the surroundings. The door to the
craft silently closed and the two walked up the road out of sight.
"Well, we have a whole day to think about what we are going to do
about acquiring this jewel we need," Slonic said.
"Well, how far is it to Ursulia?" Azul asked.
"It would take three weeks to get there by water barge and a lot
longer on horseback," Slonic scratched at his back and then started
to walk towards the riverside with Dorian and Nolon taking one last
look at the slender craft before peeling their eyes from it to
concentrate on where they were going.

Zronisk, spoke to his dark follower who had a hooded cloak, two
zombies at his side, and an undead dog on a chain its teeth yellow
with a few broken. "Find the *crimson fire gem* and the magic sword.
Bring them to me." Without a sound the follower of corruption
nodded and left the unholy church with the two walking corpses the
undead dog pulling on the chain eager to attack anything that was
alive. They went to the back of the graveyard where there was a
small craft sprayed black and entered it setting a course to Turgon
where Dorian and friends were.

Azul and Dorian sat by the evening fire and talked about whatever
came to mind. "You sure took out that troll," Dorian said
remembering the mess she had made.
"I feel a bit bad about that," she replied softly.
"But, it was going to kill us. You acted in self-defence."
"Yes, but afterwards I felt that I could have stunned it and we could
have let it live and passed by it."
"It would have probably killed others if you had let it live," Dorian
said knowing that some trolls couldn't care less about life.
"True, but I don't feel good about taking life."
"Well that means that you are a good person. At least you had the
decency to feel that way," Dorian stopped there and Azul looked
into his eyes. There was a moment of silence and they both smiled
and looked away. Slonic, came over and sat at a nearby chair.
"Where is Nolon?" Dorian asked.
"He is just outside cleaning his sword."
The two aliens that had landed earlier came into the well lit room of
the hostel dining area and stood near the bar showing cards with

pictures to communicate what they wanted. The man soon served them some ale and they continued to stand and sip at their beverages looking around.

Slonic, approached them and spoke in their language by using the *universal translator*, "Greetings there friends. How is time passing for you?"

They spoke about their travels around this part of the galaxy and finished by saying that they were doing some sightseeing on this planet. Slonic, steered the conversation towards the continent of Ursulia. They seemed interested in visiting that part of the world when Slonic described waterfalls that were over two hundred feet high and forests that had trees with leaves that glowed different colours at night amid the scents of dizzying perfumes from tropical plants. Slonic, then mentioned that they were going there and politely, the alien who's name was Lar, offered to take them first thing in the morning. Slonic, motioned with a hand for the others to come over so Nolon, followed by Azul and Dorian approached and introduced themselves. They talked for about an hour before Dorian, feeling sleepy said he was heading for the comfort of his bed. By midnight they were all asleep with the exciting prospect of flying in a space craft to the other side of the world the next day.

The silver craft was silent as it glided across the plains. Inside, it was cool and the light wasn't too bright. A sheet of toughened clear plastic composite allowed them to see out and the terrain was spectacular. Lar, deliberately didn't fly the craft too fast so that they could all admire the view. Forests swept past and rolling hills dotted with farm houses displayed the simplicity of life below. Then, they were zooming over the ocean. It was still light and Lar plunged the ship into the waters of the sea and strange fishes, octopus and the occasional whale could be seen as they slowed down to look at the majestic sealife of the world. The space craft slowly descended to the murky depths of the ocean until there was no sunlight. Lar's friend, Hom set the flash timer to blink a beam of light out in the dark and snap some pictures at the startled blind creatures that lurked down there. Hom and Lar were jittery with excitement. "We've heard that a great Yarmuth lives in these oceans. It is apparently the most shy of sea creatures, mainly feeding on plant matter and never found in the sunlit waters," Lar said. Hom, pulled open a cabinet and unhooked a pot from a rail. "You must all be hungry," he said as he began dropping pasta ringlets into the pot and filling it with water. Dorian, nodded with a rumbling in his stomach; the others agreed. They ate a typical meal from Hom and Lar's homeworld which was to the satisfaction of all new to the myriad of tastes Hom had cooked up. They stayed for about an hour with no sign of a Yarmuth, but the camera had taken some nice shots of some of the marine life. Lar, then lifted the craft out of the sea and resumed flying to Ursulia. After about half an hour Azul noticed a tentacle dangling over the clear window. "I think that there is something clinging to the ship," she said. Hom told Lar and he spun the craft around; a great octopus had attached itself to the ship while they rested under water and was refusing to let go. "There is not a lot I can do," Lar said as he resumed normal flight, "Its suckers are firmly attached to the vessel's epidermis. After about an hour they landed on a platform in a space port in Ursulia with the octopus gripping the ship. They left the ship and Hom said, "I think it is stuck to it and can't get off."

"Well," Lar said, "There is not a lot we can do." So, they left the sea creature blinking at the lights that lit up the port hoping that when they returned it would be gone. Slonic, thanked the aliens for their hospitality and Dorian, Azul and Nolon went in search of a place to stay the night.

Coruja, the owl, who is the *author of the prophecies*, was in a dream state. Though he was aware of his surroundings he had projected his inner eye to the planet Turgon. He watched Dorian as the boy walked next to Azul. The owl could hear what was being spoken and Dorian talked of his joy of being chosen to go and learn at the *castle of fateful night*. Azul, with her calm blue eyes and nice light brown skin talked about her homeworld which Dorian was surprised to learn was not Skyworld. When Azul spoke of racism towards her, because she looked different from most of the inhabitants, Dorian instantly grew angry and spoke with venom about people who were closed minded. Slonic, then said, "Dorian, joy is far from you now. Remember the lesson. Joy is much more precious than anger." Immediately, the boy calmed and tried to return to the element of joy which was much more pleasing to be with. Coruja, contemplated this for a moment before rising from his dream trance and flipping a page of the book he was reading.

The follower of darkness and corruption landed on Turgon in the Ursulia continent. A great city sprawled before him. The two zombies emerged from the craft staggering and dripping saliva from their mouths. The undead dog was on a lead and sniffed the air. They slowly walked into the night and as a few people were also about, some intoxicated while others were sitting on benches engaged with pleasant conversation, an unholy stench emanated from the undead and a few heads turned to see the follower of corruption and the undead walk by. A woman, in her forties, mocked the dark follower, just so he could hear her. He turned his head and waved his wand. Immediately the woman's nose began to bleed and her skin turned green then she began to vomit. The follower of corruption smiled and continued to walk with his loping zombies and the dog which had some of its flesh missing around his mouth so it looked like it was constantly growling.

The Lord of Death was browsing through the half price sale they had on in a shop after getting some money from the bank. There was an electronic frog whose tongue flipped out when a fly got too near, grasping it, swallowing it and excreting it in a neat little bundle. Also, there were other household items that Faramel might find useful like a cloth that cleans up stains, which was always damp and the dirt was evaporated leaving a clean smell. But, a rubbery snake, that you hold with your hand, its tongue which was as long as the snake itself was called, *dustlicker 2000*. A demonstration of the item showed that it was efficient at removing dust at an astonishing speed. The lord knew that the imp enjoyed dusting so he purchased this machine for 34 marks and had it wrapped in purple paper. Pleased that he had found something that Faramel would appreciate, he went to the card shop to buy a suitable card for his friend.

It was a cool night when Slonic pointed to a neat building tucked away between two shops that sold clothes and stationery. The facade of it was decorated in gold and scarlet; a sign hung just by the doorway which read, '*Vacancies*.' The *universal translator* also decyphered writing and they walked up the wooden steps and entered the warm hallway. Inside it was not over furnished and a man with a mild countenance greeted them. It was not long before they were shown to a pleasant room that over looked the fountain just outside and there were four beds with side tables and lamps illuminating the room. Nolon, fell onto a bed and sighed with relief at the exhaustion he felt. Azul, peered outside the window and admired the succession of street lights that ran down the road, she opened the window and a scent of lemon wafted in from the fruit trees below. The night passed fairly uneventfully and the new morning's sun's rays streamed in from the window awakening the sleepers. When they had all got dressed they descended the stairs to enter into the dining room where breakfast was being served. A fair haired man with a leather jacket sat near the window, with a visual screen in his hand, reading an article in the day's news. Dorian and Azul had a slushy cold lime drink and Nolon sipped tea with Slonic. They talked about the teachings of the Virtuous Creator and each one said a silent grateful thought for the days blessing of life as they were taught to do.

The weather was mild and a streak of grey clouds was strewn across the sky letting in, intermittently, bursts of sun as the day progressed. A miner's shop with an anvil hung above the door was what Slonic was hoping would be the place to purchase what they needed. They entered the shop and Nolon wearily hoped that the anvil was secure enough that it would not drop on him as he walked under it through the doorway. Inside, it was deep in shadow and a wooden box of rusted nails, by the door, was marked with a price for a handful. A tough man in an apron was beating a length of hot metal, sweat dripping off of his brow and he didn't stop for a few minutes though aware that customers were in his shop. The room that they were in was big enough for a troop of horsebacked riders to race around in. On the further side of the great room there stood three men in neat black chequered clothes, they had blast guns in their hands and patrolled around the more expensive items that were for sell here. A couple of elegant ladies looked at what was on display in the glass cabinets with a little boy wearing an emerald embroidered hat. Slonic, and the three walked up to see what was on display and soon found that precious stones and jewellery were in abundance held in place by pins on velvet cushions. A man with a slightly lopsided pointy nose came up to them and asked if they were looking for anything in particular. Slonic, nodded and said, "Yes. We are trying to acquire a rare stone. It is known as a *crimson fire gem* from where we come from."

"Ah yes, *asculia demeri*. We have one such jewel left over here," he motioned with his hand for them to follow as he walked to another cabinet. Pointing at a vermillion gem which sparkled in the lights that hung over head. "It is about the right size," Azul remarked to Slonic.

"Yes it is," Slonic said satisfied that it was indeed what they were looking for. "How much," he enquired.

"Its price is..." the man fumbled with an electronic device with a screen and tapped a few buttons, "4999 marks."

Slonic, was aware that it would be expensive, considering for that price one could but a hovercar for that much. He pulled out his money pouch and withdrew five thousand marks, in notes, and waited as the man unlocked the cabinet and disabled the defence grid that secured the safety of the precious gems. The man took the money and handed the open, small box to Slonic. They all admired the jewel before Slonic slipped it into his coat and they departed the shop. Outside Dorian and Nolon were with great excitement as they had succeeded in attaining what they had come here for. Slonic, gasped in pain as a zombie dog had launched itself and sunk its teeth into his calf muscle on his leg. Nolon and

Dorian, turned to see two undead and the dark follower of corruption advancing; both drew their swords. The dark follower unleashed a cackling fireball which was hurled at Dorian. It was too fast to react to but as it was about to scorch Dorian to cinders *steelfang* emanated a chime like a small bell and the assault was absorbed by the magical sword. Azul, was the next to react as Slonic drew out a dagger to deal with the dog. Her *lightning flare* flew from her fingertips directly at the dark corruptor but he managed to create a *night shield* deflecting the energy from her attack. Nolon, swung his sword into the neck of the nearest zombie and withdrew it fast enough to strike again. Slonic, managed to dispatch the unholy canine abomination and turned to face the corruptor. The follower of darkness had a knowing smile on his lips as he flung a web of *instant disintegration* towards Slonic. The defender reacted quickly, by a wave of a hand and a word, a wall of earth erupted from the ground to engulf the deadly attack. Slonic turned and with a serious warning told the three to run. Nolon had sunk his sword into the zombies repeatedly but with little effect, they were already dead and only Dorian's sword seemed to pain them. Azul, grabbed Dorian and shouted for Nolon to run. They left Slonic battling with the unholy aggressors and magic flared as each user of spells hurled offensive magic at each other.

They ran as fast as they could, Dorian fearing for Slonic's life but knew that he was skilled in combat and Azul took a last backwards glance before they turned a corner. The zombies were as fast as them but they kept on running until completely lost in the backstreets of the city. Out of breath with adrenaline surging through their veins they stopped to regain their composure. "I think we are safe," Nolon said. A few moments passed until they realized that they were on their own without the guidance of their mentor. "So what do we do now?" Azul said.

Dorian, thought about Slonic, "Shall we return to see if he is all right?"

"That could be dangerous," Nolon said.

"I think we should wait a while," Azul said, sure that Slonic would want them to be away from danger. Eventually, when their breathing returned to normal they walked out of the alleyway and into a wide street that was unfamiliar to them.

The day drew on as the three young ones walked the city not really knowing what to do. They had money in their pouches and decided to eat near the river in a small bakery that had a serving area. "I think we should return to the guest house where we slept last night. I think Slonic would expect to find us there," Dorian said as a wave of cold air blew over him.

"Yes, I think that is a good idea," Nolon acquiesced. Azul, nodded and after they had eaten they tried to find their way back to the room they had rented on the other side of the city. It took a couple of hours and night fell before they saw the familiar street where they had been staying at the house decorated in gold and scarlet. Upon walking in a waft of cooked meat stew and the clatter of cutlery being cleaned came to their awareness. Dorian and Nolon went up to their room to see if Slonic was up there and Azul went to the dining area to see if he was there. Nolon realized that they didn't have the key to the room and Azul came up moments after with it and unlocked the door. There was no sign of Slonic and the three were concerned about him theorizing that he might be dead. This brought thoughts of how they were to get back to Skyworld without him and the possibility of being stranded here, on this planet away from home, was not a pleasant thought. As the hour grew late they fell asleep and were woken by the birds singing in the morning and an angry dog barking at the passersby. During breakfast in the dining area a man with a bushy beard and a chain with various keys dangling from his belt walked in. He sat at a table and eyed the three as he ate his fried meat and drank what looked like bitter ale from a mug. "That man gives me the creeps," Azul said as she noticed a wink from the man's weathered face accompanied with a smile. Dorian looked at him and noticed a small tattoo of a serpent on his thumb and said, "He seems all right. Just another stranger." They left the building and went for a walk to where they last saw Slonic. The only signs of the struggle was a smear of blood on the ground from where the zombie dog had bitten Slonic. There were no other traces that the follower of corruption and his undead had left. "So what do we do?" Azul asked and turned to Dorian with a look of despair.

Dorian, reached into his cloak pocket and pulled out the metal box that Slonic had given him and slid the name plate. It opened and a miniature stone owl appeared wearing glasses; in front of it was a book on a lectern. After a few moments Dorian said to Azul and Nolon, "It may be able to help us if we ask the right questions."

They thought for a while until Azul said, "We're lost," to the owl. A few pages of the stone book turned and the owl spoke, "Do not fear for the Virtuous Creator and his angels are watching. Have hope that you will return to where you want to be and pray."

Nolon then said, "Yes, we haven't said a prayer for a while."

Dorian agreed, "We are supposed to pray every day and night. Maybe it is time for us to do so."

"But not here," Azul said afraid that it was the last time they saw the evil follower and that he might return.

"Okay," Dorian said and walked off toward the small park of trees just opposite the shop that sold postcards and music disks. Upon entering the park Azul began to cry. "I hope Slonic is all right."

Dorian put a reassuring arm around her and said, "We must trust in the Virtuous Creator and remember what the stone owl said about us being watched by him and his angels." Azul, wiped her tears and regained her composure. They sat down and joined hands to pray. Each said what was on their minds and gave thanks sending their love to all that are good with healing thoughts directed at the suffering. "I feel better," Azul said and the others agreed. A cloud of orange blossom swirled around them as they stood up with a scent unfamiliar to them yet pleasing. "Slonic, must be somewhere," Nolon said then he and the other two felt a sudden uneasiness. They turned and before them the follower of evil was walking towards them, alone. "Oh no!" Azul said. Dorian and Nolon drew their swords in unison. The corruptor had his hands clenched by his side and a magical fire was sparking around them ready to ignite. "What do you want?" screamed Nolon, but there came no sound from the evil man and as he advanced Nolon charged him sword in hand. Nolon, was lifted off his feet into the air and held there choking as an invisible force gripped his throat. Azul, sent a blast of energy directed at the cowled figure, but a wave of his hand rendered her attack futile. Dorian, then charged toward him wielding *steelfang*. The evil follower waved his other hand and a wall of impenetrable thorns sprung up surrounding Dorian. A cloud of fog then arose and the three students from the *castle of fateful night* fell into a sleep. When the three awoke they were in a stiflingly warm sealed room with six others who were roughly the same age. They seemed to be in a moving vehicle and through a hole in the side Dorian could see outside as the scenery passed by he knew they were going somewhere, but where? The other young ones were scared; one named Yo said that he had been a slave for three years and was now being taken to another mistress. Realizing then that they were to be sold as servants to do work the three retreated into their minds to contemplate their fate. Dorian, soon noticed that *steelfang* his magical sword was gone and the only thing he had left was the metal box with the owl. Nolon, cursed and said, "Will we ever get back to Skyworld?"

Azul, had some form of metal gloves that covered her hands and were chained together to stop her using magic. The vehicle rumbled on for what seemed an interminably long time before coming to a halt. A few moments passed until the back of the truck was opened and the prisoners were led out and into a space craft. There was not a lot they could do but ascend the ramp to the craft with various prods from a *metal electrifier* to encourage them. The craft lifted off into the late day and they were soon in space heading somewhere.

The Lord of Death sat on his throne contemplating the conference of the Lords of Mortis Divinus, which was to be held on the planet Yar Imil. There would be talk of rule over mortals and laws concerning the management of duty. The lord sat there wondering if Halorian the high wizard of Welzor will attend. He was known to provoke anger in the council and though he has a legitimate right to be within the discussions many sought his downfall, though there were rumours that the wizard had been slain. The lord's mind wandered from the television screen to the packet of crisps to the present wrapped up next to the cough sweets on the small table next to him. A man was being chased down a forest path with six pursuers brandishing clubs. He watched as the time for the man's life was running out. They caught him and beat him. One aggressor pulled out a whip which had sharp metal ends attached to the tips of the leather strands and began to use it to inflict painful wounds on the poor man. The others watched and jeered. They threw punches and kicks until the poor man was unconscious. The lord flicked a series of buttons and a menu came up explained what the man had done to deserve the scourge. According to the information the only thing the man had done was being involved in an argument with the borders of his field. Apparently, his neighbour was trying to extend his land beyond the old tree that had marked the boundaries for decades. There was a bleep and the lord watched the thugs walk away as the man's life was ended. The lord selected the one with the whip and took his identity number. Angel mice descended and the lord tapped his ring to appear there. A silvery spirit rose from the dead shell and the man looked at the angel mice as they circled around him. "So, this must be the afterlife?"

The lord replied, "An untimely death considering the potato flake is mocking the work of the giant beetle."

The man smiled and said, "I am sure I will make sense of that at some point." The angel mice wrapped invisible cords around the spirit and lifted him up, flapping their wings, he was taken to the realm to be judged.

At the *castle of fateful night* in the throne room the lord picked up his mobile phone which he seldom used. Tapping a few numbers he was put through to Juiz the rat. "I have another assignment for you. The number is 9845798. Make sure you make him choke on the holy smoke of a decaying weevil."

Juiz, replied by saying that justice will be done, and wondered what victim was next before leaving for his job.

A flying arachnid landed on Zronisk's shoulder. "Ah, *creepwing.* You have something for me." Wrapped in a silky embrace on the creature's leg there was a small metal tube. Zronisk took it and slid it in to a small viewing machine. An image was projected into the air and Groni's image appeared; he spoke, "Darkness forever!!" came the salute. "I have found some new information about the *crown of death.* As I had thought it requires eleven stones to be fully operational." He went through the list of gems that were needed and then said," I warn you not to use it until it is working properly because it will degrade the power in the other stones. Also, I have found out that there is a deadly disease being held within the power of the crown. It has something to do with the stability of the universal jewel of sadness. The jewel can only operate with this deadly infectious virus."

Zronisk, looked at the crown and realized that two of the other jewels' lights had gone out. Groni continued, "There is no known cure for the deadly disease and it has been known to infect and destroy great nations of other worlds." Groni's, voice took on a tone of amusement and Zronisk immediately thought of how he could control such a devastating natural virus.

"So, Groni continued, "You need to recover the other gems to fix the crown," Groni, smirked and then said, "May nightmares abound and haunt the followers of virtue." With that said his image fizzled out and Zronisk was now contemplating how he could turn the disease into a weapon that would destroy his enemies.

There was a bright flare of light just outside the window and the master of corruption looked out to see his follower had returned from Turgon. Within a matter of minutes the cowled figure of the follower of corruption entered the unholy church and stood before Zronisk a whisper of breath escaped his twisted mouth and he held out the *crimson fire gem.* The dark corruptor took it and with eyes glittering scrutinized it. The follower then held out *steelfang.* Slipping the jewel into his cloak pocket Zronisk took the sword and ran his fingertips along the length of the blade. There was a sharp pain as a burst of magic shot in to his hand. He dropped the weapon and cursed. "It has been infused with *sparks of virtue,*" he kicked the sword away and it slid under a wooden bookcase, "Useless," he exclaimed.

A singing sound came from the lower catacombs and Zronisk thought to himself that the prisoner needed to be tortured more to keep him quiet so he quickly made his way down the flight of stone steps and the singing continued. Entering into a room where there was a cage and a solitary prisoner singing a hymn to the Virtuous Creator seemed most jubilant. "I've told you about this before,"

Zronisk said. "You know how it irritates me when I am trying to think."

The man, in rags, replied, "I feel the need to praise our Creator and at times to pray for your soul because you are lost."

"Oh, rubbish," Zronisk said and the man burst in to song again. "You will never learn will you ?" The evil corruptor then set the straw in the cage on fire and the man yelped in pain. "That's better," Zronisk said, "I much prefer you in pain than prancing around in joy."

The fire had stopped and the man rubbed his feet and looked up, "He will forgive you, you know. Just repent and be truly sorry for all the evil you have done."

The evil corruptor shook his head sadly, "I don't think you understand the power I have and enjoy. I am not going to serve your god when I can have untold of power and glory."

"The power you have only brings misery. I fear that you have been corrupted to the point of destroying the sparks of virtue within you. You are truly lost and I see your fate will be condemnation in a fire that is unquenchable," the man had sorrow in his eyes.

"My fate is supreme. I will one day be amongst the pantheon of deities as a super power... It has been promised," Zronisk, turned and before he walked away he said, "No singing!" He paced out of the room and up the stairs and was just about to close the wooden door when he heard his prisoner burst in to song again, "I've got to do something about this," he said under his breath, "It's driving me mad."

The space craft was an old model and shaked with the movement through space until it reached a point when it became calm again and the rattling stopped. Azul, turned her blue eyes towards Dorian and said, "I think that boy is in a lot of pain," she said pointing to a young lad that had his hands wrapped around his legs and was shaking. Dorian, went up to him and asked if he was all right. The boy didn't answer and there was blood seeping through his shirt on his back. "Let me look at your wounds. I might have something that could help."

The boy unclasped his hands and said something that Dorian could barely hear. Azul, came over and lifted the shirt up and they could see that the whip had done some damage to his skin. Dorian, pulled out some herbs from his pouch with a little bottle of liquid. He began to mix them together in the palm of his hand before applying it to the rough cuts the metal tipped whip had inflicted. The boy cringed and Dorian said that the pain would soon go away. Along with the herbs and liquid Dorian said an incantation which sent a glow from his hand and the inflammation of the wounds eased.

Azul and Dorian then sat back down next to Nolon and they could see that the boy had stopped shaking.

A man came into the room with a bag of bread rolls and handed them out to the prisoners, then left without a word. They all sat in the dimly lit room chewing on the bread and afterwards Azul fell asleep leaning on Dorian so he wrapped his arm around her daring not to fall asleep in case danger presented itself.

Juiz, the rat, arrived on another planet to execute justice. He found his way to a house located in the heart of a dirty city and knocked on the door. The man that was to be judged opened the door and scowled down at the finely dressed rat and spat to his left. "What do you want you oversized vermin?" he said.

Juiz, whipped out the hand wallet and flipped it open saying, "Preordained by death." As he said the words he showed the badge of the insignia of the *castle of fateful night*, with an owl reading a book. The man's eyes glanced at it and there was a flash; in an instant the nasty man had lost his sight. Surprised, he stumbled and said, "What's happened?" And, regaining his balance by resting a hand on the door frame he rubbed his eyes to see but the only thing in his sight was the after impression of the owl.

Juiz, walked away without giving the man an answer. There would be another cheque coming his way for the work he had done and justice has been achieved.

Awaking in a room with the scent of medicine, Slonic lifted his head and felt the pain on his chest. He remembered then. The follower of corruption had caught him off guard and had blasted him with a deadly spell that would have been fatal if he hadn't deflected some of it with his defensive magic. His hand immediately went for where the gem was, but it was gone. "I see you are awake," a voice came from a middle aged woman who walked up to him and smiled. "You are in the care of healers. You were found unconscious, lying in the street. Morisu found you and you have been here for about sixteen hours."

"That long," and Slonic lifted himself up, wincing. "I need to get out of here," he said and swung himself off the bed. His clothes were folded on a chair next to the bed and he began to dress.

"I would advise that you at least have something to eat before you go," the woman then said, "Down the hallway to the left. That's were the kitchens are. I'm sure you'll find something that will suffice you for your travels."

Slonic, walked out and took the nurse's advice heading for the canteen.

The craft took what seemed like days to finally reach its destination. A bright sun greeted the captives as they were led out of the craft and shepherded into a vehicle that was stuffy and smelt foul. The man, that Dorian had seen at the guest house with the tattoo of a snake on his hand, was puffing a pipe and his six henchmen poked the young ones until they were all loaded in the truck. Azul, gave a look of disgust at the smoking man before the back hatch was sealed shut and they were on their way to a destination that all were dreading. Inside, Nolon was in a dire mood because he no longer had his sword that he surmised must have been taken by the captors. Dorian, wondered if his father would be angry that he had lost *steelfang* and he hoped that he would recover it one day, if he survived his captivity. Azul, had tried to slip the metal gloves off from her hands so she could cast spells again for she had tried summoning magic but with no success.

The truck rumbled across a muddy trail through a flat landscape that had fields of grain growing and as Dorian peered through a rusty crack in the vehicles side he knocked his head as the wheel hit a ditch and jolted everyone. "What are we going to do?" Azul said hoping for an answer that would ease her worried mind.

"Well," Dorian said, "When we get to where we are going then we can make an escape plan.

"As long as we are not split up," Nolon said.

"If I can get these gloves off," Azul tried again to prize the strap off, "They won't stand a chance."

"We'll find a way," Dorian said reassuringly.

"I wonder what planet we're on. We must be miles away from home. And, how are we going to get back?" Nolon, looked at the others in the same predicament. They were not much older than himself and they had families; others that would be concerned and fretful about their safety.

Time passed slowly until the truck eventually came to a halt. There was a moment of stillness then the bar from the back of the vehicle was lifted and daylight streamed in. Dorian shielded his eyes and a gruff voice ordered them to exit the truck. They all stood and stepped out into daylight. It took a few moments for their eyes to adjust to the brightness, then they could see the orange bricked building that loomed against clear blue sky. In single file they were led to the structure and they entered it. The man with the serpent tattoo was nowhere to be seen, but a few of the other men with electrifying rods prodded their prisoners with sharp jolts of energy to make them move faster. Inside, they were led to a large room where there were rows of bunk beds, each had a number on them. They were handed scraps of paper saying which bed was to be theirs and Azul cringed as a beetle scurried down the wall and under one of the blankets. They were left in that room for hours and they all talked among themselves. One of the younger girls whose name was Armina was constantly in tears and her brother tried to ease her sorrow by promising that they would all be all right.

When night fell four men came into the room and told them that they had to start work. This made them apprehensive as to what this was going to be. They were led down several corridors then into a huge room with machinery. There were others there operating the machines and some were sewing, and sealing boxes up. Nolon, was taken to be trained on a plastic former, which shaped plastic to specific contours. Azul, with her gloves on was taken to the kitchens to wash up and clean. Dorian, was told to sweep the floor of the factory which took over two hours. Their work went on deep in to the hours of the night and anyone caught falling asleep was prodded with the *electrifier*. When the dawn sun arose a loud whistle blew and they were allowed to return to their sleeping quarters. Slumping down on his bed Dorian feared that he would never leave this awful place and then remembered to have hope. His thoughts became calm and his faith was strengthened. He pulled out the metal box and slid the name plate; the owl was revealed. He spoke softly to it saying, "A lesson on virtue and corruption." The owl began to read and speak from the book of Everlasting Truths:

"A darkness corrupt hidden in virtue and a virtue manifest hidden in corruption."

"Beware, for if you are attracted by virtue there may be a spark of corruption hidden within. The followers of evil hide their distortions in virtue so as to attract and deceive the innocent towards the nature of evil. They try all ways of trickery so as to corrupt and will persuade you to corruption by using examples that are misleading."

"By perfection of the four spiritual skills that allow one to see, feel, hear and know energy will you be better prepared to uncover any deception."

"Also, by studying the book of everlasting truths will you be better able to defend yourselves against any corruption and will also allow you to enhance your virtuous nature so as to become incorruptible."

"By the nature of things virtue can be obscured by the darkness of corruption, so always be careful and attentive of your judgements on discerning good from evil. For, the followers of corruption will hide from you a fellow being of goodness that is in need. Because the book of Everlasting Truths teaches not to reward evil, you must be aware that there may be many occasions which must be attended to when someone requires your aid and they may seem evil but are in truth shrouded with darknesses to deceive anyone virtuous so as not to assist. It is sad to say that some are neglected because they are thought evil."

"Once again to learn the four spiritual skills of perception will allow you to see into the true meaning and character of things."

After the lesson Dorian closed the metal box and hid it in his cloak hoping that it would go undiscovered.

Zronisk, the dark follower of corruption went to pick up the *crown of death* and a blackish purple mist seeped out of it giving a warm sensation on his hand. It billowed in the air and dispersed. "Odd," he thought and placed the crown on his head to see if it would actually work this time. A sound of thousands of people screaming filled his head and grew in intensity. Zronisk, enjoyed the screaming for it was his sort of thing but it eventually got to the point it was so loud that he instantly received a pounding headache. Taking the crown off he decided to visit his prisoner to take out his frustration on him. Descending the steps and walking into the chamber of torture he was greeted with a scene that brought great anger and rage to him. Before him was his favourite zombie on his knees praying. "I've converted him to the Virtuous Creator," the prisoner said. Although in a cage he had managed to persuade the zombie of the importance of prayer and repentance. So, the zombie, though having some intelligence and being animated decided to risk a prayer. Zronisk, slapped the undead male out of his reverent prayer and ordered it to lick the floor. He left then and expected the floor to be shining upon his return. "I will deal with you later," he snapped at the prisoner as he turned to leave.

The conference of the Lords of Mortis Divinus was being held in the *sacred tower of the elementals*. A magnificent room hosted the event and twenty one Lords of Death were seated around a massive circular table which was made of precious stones; in the centre, there was depicted a four headed dragon breathing fire upon an army of lizardmen. The Lord of Death from the *castle of fateful night* was the last to arrive and sat himself upon a silver chair studded with curls of sea shells. One tall lord then greeted the council, "My friends from the realms of the universe, thank you for attending this conference. As you all well know we have a lot to discuss. But, first we will start with a round and an update on what has been concerning you or things needed to be taken into consideration." He sat back down and in a clockwise fashion, one by one each lord stood and informed the council of news. The lord from the *castle of fateful night* was busy playing, 'Knock out the Troll,' on his Zorgamez consol. When it finally came to him to talk he slouched back in the chair and muttered something about, "Fire stalks run around causing porridge to dance upon twisted forks." Only the lead lord of death found him amusing and he said, "Yes, we will return to you regarding the prophecy later.."

Slonic, had eaten and was now fumbling in his side pack and pulled out a small device that looked like a golden nugget with a few buttons on it. He pressed on a small nodule and a screen appeared in mid air. It was a tracking device and was homing in on the metal box which taught from the book of Everlasting Truths that Dorian had. It was a precaution he had taken, just in case they got separated. There was a solar system and the arrow pointed to a planet. 'Not too far away then,' he thought, as it was near this planet and not across the other side of the galaxy.

It was the afternoon when they were served the first meal of the day. Nolon, spooned the thick soup into his mouth and was one of the quickest to finish. "I wonder what we are going to do today?"
Dorian, said that they were probably going to go to the factory and he dreaded sweeping floors again. After their lunch the guards came and took them to the work floor where others were already busy doing jobs. The hours seemed to drag by as Dorian was given task after task. It was quite gloomy in the room and Dorian was told to watch the lamps and to refill them with oil when the flames extinguished. A woman with long black hair and blue eyes walked around with the man with the serpent tattoo and she observed them all with their labour. Dorian, noticed that she was watching him and saw her point at him and talk to the man whose name Dorian didn't know but because of his tattoo Azul had named him *Viper*. Before the hour had passed Dorian was summoned and taken to another room where a desk and piles of papers were stacked high. In the room *Viper* was there with the woman, he said, "It looks like it's your lucky day. You will be going with Miss Vober to work for her. Consider yourself honoured for she has chosen you to go with her today. Dorian, looked at her; she came over and jabbed a pin into his arm which made him yelp in pain. "Why did you do that?" Dorian asked angrily.
"Don't you dare speak to me in that tone of voice," she said as if

every word she uttered were an order she was so used to give and it was always obeyed.

Dorian, didn't say a word and she smiled a most loathsome smile with her black lipstick that made her look like someone that could poison you with a spoken word. "Answer me!" she snapped.

Dorian wasn't about to say sorry and he controlled his anger and said, "Nothing is hidden from the Virtuous Creator."

The colour drained from her face and then she laughed a most wicked sound, "The darkness is stronger. You will learn to appreciate that fact and I think I am going to enjoy breaking you."

Viper, sat amused at the woman. He respected her and knew she was evil but there was something fascinating about her that made him admire her. "Your zip car is here," he said as he saw the hover car come to a halt outside.

Dorian, didn't have a choice. He was led to the transportation and felt a pang of loss thinking of Azul and Nolon. They would be wondering what would happen to him and he didn't dare ask to go the retrieve his cloak with the metal box and herb pouches.

The choir was assembled and the three followers of darkness with Zronisk looked upon them with satisfaction. There were eleven zombies in all and bits of decaying matter would fall off their skin as they stood their awaiting instructions. Zronisk spoke, "On this dark evening we will sing, 'Decay and be glad,' a song from olden times and one that will give our god of corruption great pleasure as we lower our voices to sing his praise." And Zronisk began, "O rot and filth decay.. We praise our god decay... " The zombies made the most awful noise. They were all out of tune and during the recital one would pause and retch throwing sick all over the place. A hand dropped off during the words, "Fill us with power to fulfil your darkest plans..." A rat was nibbling at one of the undead's feet and Zronisk encouraged them to sing louder relishing in the disharmony. They sang a few more songs with words from their unholy book which was called, the *ultimate book of power and corruption*. During the performance Zronisk, the dark master, had a tape recording of it and later on in the evening he sat with a glass of alcoholic milk listening to the wailing through some headphones. His smile was one of reverence and pride, he knew that the dark one would appreciate the fine qualities of the undead choir, thinking this as he tapped his foot to the non existent rhythm.

When the day shift was over and they were allowed a break Azul was concerned that there was no sign of Dorian. A boy called Horanthian said that he saw Dorian being taken away in a zip car and that he was with the mistress Vober. "She is an evil woman and worships the dark corruptor," he shivered as he mentioned her name and said that she lived on the other side of the great lake. Nolon and Azul talked of how to get out of this predicament that they were in and they formed a plan. There was a machine in the work room that was used to cut sheets of strengthened plastic. Azul, said that they might be able to use it to free her of the metal gauntlets she was wearing and therefore she would be able to cast spells. "After our night shift we can sneak in and try to use the machine to break the fastenings on your gloves," Nolon suggested. Azul, agreed and said, "We could free the others as well. This is no place for us or them." Nolon, acquiesced and said that we will also need a space faring vessel to get off this planet. That will be difficult because we will need to find someone with the skills not to mention acquiring a ship." This left them thinking and an hour passed before they were led again to the work place to continue their unpaid labour.

Dorian, had a ball and chain attached to his ankle. He found it difficult cleaning the vast tiled floor that looked clean before he started but mistress Vober would point out smears that were invisible to the eye and snap at him making him feel like whatever he did he did wrong. Dorian, worked for hours at a time and his arms were tired and sore. He would stop for a few moments to ease his pain but was constantly aware that she could appear at any moment so he rested when absolutely necessary. The floor, as far as Dorian could tell, was spotless and when miss Vober didn't come to inspect it he waited until the clock rang out midnight. He wasn't sure what to do so he went to his room which was with the animals in the stable. He had a blanket and no pillow. Within moments he fell asleep until a bucket of cold water was thrown over him with miss Vober standing there scowling at him, "Who told you you could go to sleep? Come on get up. Just one more job to be done then you can rest."
He arose and walked with her to the kitchens. There was a great pile of dirty dishes to wash up and he set upon this task listlessly and apathetically. He was alone for about an hour and a half before it was all done and had not eaten for many hours. Before leaving for the stable he took a peek inside the cupboard for a crust of bread and found a plate of pastries. Taking three of them he ate them as fast as possible before anyone found out and walked back to where he was to sleep dragging the iron ball that caused great discomfort. Inside the stable he lit a small plate with herbs on to make the smell not so bad and knelt down to pray. He prayed to the Virtuous Creator, telling him of his despair and worries and before finishing he wished a kiss to find its way to Azul from him.

That night he dreamed of Azul's bright blue eyes.

At the conference of the Lords of Mortis Divinus there was an air of anticipation as the Lord from the *castle of fateful night* stood to address those assembled to give a report of his dealings with mortals. "I have squiggled the crushed mushroom and in due time the hair of the imperial sprout will grow," he seemed satisfied that he had said all that was necessary and sat back down. There were a few chuckles and another lord stood and said, "Your report was unsatisfactory."

The lord of death from the Octopus galaxy then stood and said, "Yes, it seems that the prophecy needs to be fulfilled."

Another then said, "I understand that one has been chosen?"

There were a few whisperings and Octavis the grand Lord of Death spoke saying, "A boy called Dorian has been selected to replace the current lord. He is unfit to rule... as you can tell..."

There followed a brief amount of chattering and a Lady Death stood and said, "It seems unfair that the Lord from Skyworld should be replaced. After all we know his crown has been degraded and it is only a matter of time that the jewels will be replaced." A few muttered in agreement but the grand Lord of Death spoke next, "The thing is even when the gems are replaced there remains the fact that his mind has been damaged and it will leave psychological scarring. He will never be the same again. The kindest thing we can do is to allow the transformation process to work and to allow Dorian the ceremony of Fearsome Divinity to take place."

The Lady Death sat back down to contemplate the words of the grand Lord of Death. The conference continued and covered dimensional matters as well as evil incarnations that was a key concern to the debate, yet the mind of the lord from Skyworld was not really paying attention to the matters.

It was Faramel's birthday and the Lord of Death had arrived back from the conference. He had three hours before Faramel was due to return from a visit to his parents who lived on another world. So, the lord decided to make a cake. He used pineapple jam and decorated the topping with chopped nuts. It looked like a sad thing that needed to be eaten rather quickly so as to put it out of its misery. But, the lord was quite pleased for he hadn't made a cake for over a thousand years. Waiting patiently on his throne he watched an episode of Goblin Greed, a comedy involving a greedy goblin and his friends that get up to mischief in a castle owned by a vampire that was afraid of the dark. He watched on with amusement until Faramel arrived carrying an armful of presents. "Happy Birthday!" the lord said, happy to see the imp.

"You remembered!" the imp said happily.

"Yes, and I have a present for you," the lord handed Faramel the present. The imp was most impressed and unwrapped it with vigour.

"Oh, brilliant. I heard these are really good," he said holding out the snake, *dustlicker 2000*.

"You can put it on automatic to clean ceilings," the lord said, "And it is supposed to be the fastest snake available.

Faramel, smiled and said that it would come in handy. "And," the lord continued, "Wait there." He returned with a cake; a solitary green candle lit upon it. The Lord of Death broke into song and sang happy birthday. Faramel, admitted that this birthday was one of his best and after cake he went for a shower in a state of joy.

It was now early afternoon and Dorian was sweeping the ground by the swimming pool that was occupied with sharks. He took a look at the deadly predators and was soon called to feed them by throwing buckets of whale and seal meat. The sharks fed in a frenzy tearing apart their food and consuming all that they had been given. When the task was done mistress Vober summoned him to a room where he had not been and was led there by To'neem a male servant. Upon entering the room miss Vober sat by a desk, she looked up and there was no trace of a smile or any goodness. "Dorian," she said, "I want to make you a follower of corruption."

At the mention of this he went pale and didn't say a word. *"Well speak then!"* she snapped.

"I have no desire to follow such an evil deity," he said knowing that to cross Miss Vober was as dangerous as standing too close to the sharks.

"Well whether you like it or not I am going to teach you to follow his will and to please him or else you will not live to see your next birthday," she stood up and grabbed his wrist digging her nails in and leading him out of the room. They passed many doors until finally coming to a locked door ornamented with symbols. She unlocked it and dragged Dorian inside. It was dimly lit and stank with putrid death. There was an altar stained with dried blood and a dead sacrificed animal was rotting upon it. Statues of unwholesome figures were in the act of doing unspeakable crimes. A rug with runes and symbols relating dark sayings was spread out and mistress Vober told him to sit down on it. "For now you will spend an hour each day in here reading from this book," she handed him a copy of the dark sayings of the evil one. "I will return shortly and if you haven't memorized six verses you will be punished," she lit a twisted candle and set it next to him on a table. The door was shut and Dorian could hear the key turning and the lock snapping into place. There was something eerie about the room, it was as if there was an unholy presence that whispered and gave life to a myriad of voices just too faint to make out what was being said. Dorian, sat on the rug and placed his hands together saying a prayer to the Virtuous Creator. His mind was troubled for when he was concentrating on the words to say a disturbing background noise was trying to distract him. Apart from tortured voices a music of disharmony was accompanying them. Time went by very slowly and Dorian could smell smoke. He opened his eyes and the room was on fire. Somehow, the candle had fallen and had set everything alight. He stood up and there was nothing he could do. Grabbing the door handle he tried to open the door as the smoke was filling the room. It was frightening that he thought he was going to die in this room but something cracked and the door opened. Leaving quickly he made his way to the outside to breathe some clean air. To'neem, noticed that Dorian was coughing and came over saying, "I thought you were in the room of the corruptor?"

Dorian, explained about the fire and To'neem said that the mistress will be very angry and it would be better not to be alive when she finds out. The servant then gathered some others to help put out the fire. Miss Vober's voice could be heard screaming as she walked down the hallway. She came out into the back garden where Dorian was sitting and grabbed him by the ear, "You've got a lot of explaining to do!" She led him to the swimming pool where the sharks were lurking underwater. "I know the Ultimate Corruptor taught us to lie," she said, "But, I want the truth! Did you set the room on fire on purpose?"

Dorian, didn't know what to say and stumbled over his words, "Um, I said a prayer and when I opened my eyes the room was on fire."

"And who did you say the prayer to? It better have not been your God!"

Dorian, knew he was in trouble and said, "Yes, but I didn't start the fire on purpose!"

Miss Vober shook him and said, "You've not only offended my dark god but you have also destroyed my sanctuary. You're of no use," she said and pushed him into the pool. Standing there to watch him being torn apart by the sharks she waited for his blood to darken the water. She waited but the sharks didn't attack, in fact they moved away from him as if he was of no interest. Mistress Vober watched on in anticipation but nothing happened. Dorian, dragged the heavy metal ball attached to the chain to the shallow end of the pool and daring not to get out and confront miss Vober he felt safer in a swimming pool of sharks. He thought he would be dead by now but for some reason the creatures were not interested in him. It seemed that the sharks were avoiding him, not even getting too close.

The insidious disease from the *crown of death* had been released and its first victim was Zronisk. A blemish appeared on his skin and boils were evident causing the master of darkness to scratch at it and it was slowly spreading. The malign power of the disease would increase in strength when it touches fire. The black mist coursed its way with the wind and grew in size scattering its tendril like wisps into the breaths of farmers and any living thing. In a matter of days it had spread and multiplied so as to cause crops to wilt and whither. People were getting sick. It was getting stronger, parts of it had passed through fire and had become more potent. At this stage the affect it had on a local business man was immediate. He coughed and spat blood, collapsing to the ground to the horror of his colleagues. They tried to lift his head and get him to drink some cool water but his teeth were loosened and three of them fell from his jaw and clattered on the stone floor. "It's a plague," one screamed. They left him there, afraid to get too close and his skin ripped open with sore wounds exposed to the air. A man who was a follower of the Virtuous Creator, sat by him and consoled him with words that were a great comfort, but his life was slipping away. "What's happening to me?" the victim asked.

"I think that your time has come. You will be in the land of spirits soon. There will be no pain."

He rubbed his cheek and felt wet life blood smear his fingers. His wife was soon at his side and she wept. The last words that came from his lips were, "My love.. Take care of little Ella and Jon.. Tell them I love them and don't forget to kiss them for me.."

He went limp and the colour of his skin turned pale and there was no warmth left in him. His loyal wife shook with grief and her tears fell on his face as if they were both crying. The man who had sat there unafraid of any consequences that what had taken the unfortunate man might affect him, clasped his hands he spoke a prayer while the woman was crying with unhappiness. Afterwards, when many moments had passed the man stood and said, "It is probably better if his body is burnt to stop the evil from spreading. He wanted to take her hand and lead her out of the room away from the sorrow of her love, but she clinged to her dead husband and refused to leave him, without saying a word he left her there and went to get the local guard and instruct him that another victim has succumbed to the disease. In time his body will be set alight and the sadness with be in the hearts of his friends and family.

Morcego, the sneaky bat had overheard snippets of conversations at the *castle of fateful night* and Zronisk had sent his followers of corruption after the other jewels so as to complete the *crown of death*. At the moment his hand was sore and he constantly scratched it. He had sent one of his zombies down to the local apothecary to buy some cream and had written a note for zombies aren't that good at talking. The zombie had sauntered off to the high street at a loping pace. Dogs, came up to it and sniffed, some barked but the zombie ambled on in disinterest. Upon reaching a row of shops he saw a sign with a pair of healing hands held over a sick woman. He entered the shop and the sweet scent of herbs and soothing chemicals could be smelt, though the zombie didn't appreciate this and soon his over powering stink choked everyone in the room. He walked upto the counter and pulled out the handwritten note that Zronisk had made slipping it onto the counter for the young man to read. "So, you want some soothing balm?" the man said looking over his spectacles.

The zombie replied by uttering , "Yeahump."

The man then turned around and examined the rows of medicines that were available. Eventually, he picked up a tube of cream and turned back again. "I think this will do the trick," he placed the cream on the counter and said, "It is good for burns and irritations."

The zombie looked down at it and his eye fell out of his socket and landed on the counter, then it rolled off but the young man was quick and caught it. Handing the zombie back his eye, and the undead man placed it back in; he turned to leave. "Can I get you anything for your eye?"

The undead male dropped a few coins on the counter's surface and nodded. The man had seen undead before and didn't want to question him or his necromancer who had raised him might take offense. It was all too dangerous to inquire in to these things. "We have some strong glue that could work," he shuffled his feet and plucked out a small tube from an open cabinet. "The money covers the cream and the glue." The zombie than leaned over and caught his eyeball squeezed some of the super strength glue on it and then popped it back in. "It will take a few minutes to stick," the young man said.

The undead man waited a few minutes and then bent over, the eye stayed in place. The zombie smiled and a tooth fell out. "Well, you've got enough glue for your teeth as well." The zombie left leaving his tooth on the counter and the young man who served him was glad to be of assistance.

Slonic, went to the space port to hire a craft and after he had signed all the relevant documents he sped off into the night fairly confident that he could control the ship for he had been trained on using similar vessels before. Into space he went and headed for the solar system in the Thurgoni constellation. Thurgoni, was a god of dwarves and this particular planet he was heading to was known to the dark gods. He read as much as he could about life on this world known as Yeminora and there were many pictures of statues and shrines devoted to the Utimate Corruptor. This, sent an uncomfortable chill around him and he hoped that the three were still alive and well, though he felt in his heart that their lives were being watched over by the Virtuous Creator. He prayed and received an answer. The answer was to land near the *river of departed souls*. This river was named after a great battle where the slain had littered the waters and had drifted down and out to sea. There were paintings and poems about it and the more he researched the more afraid he became for them. It was not a world where the followers of virtue should ever go.

It was night and Azul, Nolon and Horanthian sneaked out of their room after picking the lock of the door which Nolon managed with a piece of wire. They walked up the main hall on soft steps being cautious and listening out for any signs of life. There were some rooms that were still lit and there were a few men throwing dice and waging bets on outcomes. The door to the factory work place was locked and after several attempts with the wire it refused to unlock. "What do we do now?" Horanthian said in a low voice. Nolon, stepped back and then lunged forward with a kick that split the door from the frame. "It's open now!" he said.
They had to be quick in case anyone had heard the break in. The machine was still plugged in and a flick of a switch activated it. "Be careful," Horanthian said to Azul. The machine blade vibrated and it made a loud noise. Three men from the previous room came in and shouted, "What do you think you're doing?" One said. At this point Azul had sheared off the clasps that held her gauntlets on; her hands were free so she could use spells. A man with a whip advanced with a crack on the floor as the metal tips hit the ground in a threatening manner. Nolon and Horanthian had no weapons but were prepared to use their fists. A man with a thin nose and black beard went to grab Nolon by the throat but Azul let forth a *stream of fire* from her fingers. The man instantly ignited and screamed. As this happened the male with the whip lashed out and caught Horanthian with the metal tips across the face and drew blood. The boy took a step back and then ran out of sight. They didn't know what to do with the man on fire as he screamed running to find the hose pipe in the garden to dowse himself. Whether he made it to the water or not they never knew. Azul warned the other men that if they continued to attack they would both end up on fire. They weren't scared by her threats and as the man with the whip

drew back his arm to send stinging lashes at them. Azul blasted a stream of fire at them both. The sound of screaming filled the air; Nolon and Azul ran back to their sleeping quarters. Once there they woke up the others and said that they were leaving this place and anyone who wanted to go with them had to leave now. Nolon, took Dorian's cloak and herb pouches and five of the young ones decided that they wanted to risk leaving with them. Any door that was locked was either kicked open or burnt down with a spell. They were in the gardens and the dogs were loose. Azul, felt bad about killing the animals so she used a sleeping spell to keep them out of action. Men could be heard yelling and the lights were turned on which lit up the grounds, though by this time they were floating up over the wall with a levitation spell from Azul. "Hey! Wait for me!" came Horanthian's voice as he came running up. They were glad to see him and before long all eight were on the other side and heading across open ground. "Do you think they will follow us?" Azul said a little out of breath.

"Yeah, or who else would do their dirty work," Nolon said bitterly.

"We must find Dorian," Azul stated.

Horanthian led the way with a wary eye behind him for he knew it wouldn't be long before they were hounded down. Nolon, could see in the distance a row of trees and Horanthian said that the lake was past the trees. Mistress Vober lives just beyond the lake and it would take a couple of hours to get there. They kept walking at a brisk pace until, looking behind them, they could see lights bobbing up and down as the men from the work house were giving them chase.

Zronisk, went down to the lower chambers of the unholy church to torment his prisoner, but he was gone and had left a note. It read: I've tried to plant a seed of faith in your heart but it withered. There may come a time when you renounce your evil ways but I fear that it will never happen for you are truly tainted and fully corrupted. I have pity on your soul and I pray that you will not suffer the neverending pain in damnation but I am not sure that you will change. May the glorious Creator watch over you, *Truliaron*. Zronisk, screwed up the bit of paper in his hand and threw it in the air where it ignited and fell to the floor burning. He cursed his prisoner and wondered how he had managed to get away, the door to his cage was firmly locked and as far as he knew he didn't know magic. "Well," he thought, "I'll just have to get some other follower of the Virtuous Creator to torture." Just after this thought he heard the space craft land outside, and the other corruptors he had sent to retrieve the jewels had returned. There was also someone knocking on the door but he ignored it and went out the back to see if his followers had been successful in getting the precious gemstones. The door to the craft slid open and the followers of corruption emerged. They walked up to their master and presented him with the other jewels that were needed for the *crown of death*. Zronisk, was overcome with glee and took the gems into the building and went to get the crown. There was another series of knocks on the door before it was blown off its hinges with a blast spell from Groni the goblin. He stormed in and said, "Doesn't anyone answer the door round here?"

Zronisk, said that he didn't hear it and his other followers were going a bit deaf. "Anyway," he said. "You are just in time. We have all the gemstones and now I will have ultimate power over knowing the thoughts of all men."

It was night and Dorian was tied to a post and his shirt was ripped off of him. A man with a twisted nose and curved lips lashed out with a leather strap with studs embedded within it. Dorian let out screams every time the torture weapon ripped his skin. He was sore and bleeding and it seemed to go on for hours. Mistress Vober stood and watched with satisfaction. After the punishment was finished his body was rubbed down with vinegar and salt which left him stinging. He was barely conscious and his head sagged as he hung there. Everything was a blur and Miss Vober said something to him that he couldn't make out. They left him in agony and the cold wind stung his exposed flesh. Mistress Vober walked back to her private quarters where she sat at a table and wrote out a letter to her cousin who lived on another world. She wrote of the boy Dorian and that she would be sending him to her. Her sister's name was called Hellina and she ate human flesh. 'At least he will be of some use,' miss Vober thought to herself, and Dorian would soon be off her hands, 'He is more trouble than it is worth. No one burns down my shrine to the Ultimate Corruptor and lives. Though he will be tortured to his life's end, but not quite the end," she thought about that and smiled. 'Oh what a pleasant day to please the dark one.'

Though Dorian was semi conscious he had been saying a prayer over and over again, "Please Holy Father, make the pain go away. Help me so that I do not die and will live again to see Azul," he begged and pleaded. The man with the leather strap returned and continued beating him, but for some reason Dorian could not feel any pain. He looked up at the man and and almost smiled, but dared not to. Mistress Vober then came out of the house with a small cushion which had hundreds of pins stuck in it. She proceeded to stick each one into his skin, and grew angry when Dorian didn't cry of scream. He could not feel any pain and he thanked the Virtuous Creator. When she had finished she whispered in his ear and said, "You will be taken to my sister Hellina who will cook you up and serve you for supper and what remains will be used for sandwiches for the next three days."

Dorian, knew that she was trying to frighten him and the thought crossed his mind to spit on her face but he knew that was not his way, instead he managed a weak smile and said, "You will surely pay the price for your cruelness. One day you will surely be cursed."

She laughed at him and said, "Your Virtuous Creator cannot harm me. The dark one is much more powerful, if only you'd see that you would be blessed with knowledge that will make your enemies fear you. Knowledge that will allow you to torture and kill anyone that stands against you."

Dorian, didn't reply, he felt weak and it would be futile to argue with someone that was clearly overcome with hatred and darkness. She left him to think over her words and went to the gallery where she liked to see the collection of paintings that represented horrors and unspeakable acts. With a glass of wine she walked around viewing the pictures and admiring the brush strokes and keen of eye that it took to make such works of art.

The young ones made their way around the lake when Nolon stopped and turned to look behind him. A dog jumped for his throat and he knocked it aside. Azul, turned and cast a spell on the dog and it fell asleep. The others had stopped too and then the men came into view with lanterns. They looked at each other and one man said, "You'd better come with us or you can die out here."

Azul, spoke up, "We aren't going with you. Either you return peacefully or you will be set on fire." It was only one of the few offensive spells she knew. Though she also had the power to take life she didn't feel right about it. The men laughed and one said, "You are a bit too sure of yourself. We are five and you are only children." Then one of the men went to grab Molil. He kicked and screamed for the man to let him go and that is when Azul made a venomous snake coil around his neck and bite deeply into the man's throat. He cursed and let go of the boy, wrestling with the slithery snake. He soon fell to the ground paralysed. The other that had been pursuing them took a moment to think then one raised a crossbow and took aim at Azul but she waved a hand and plants grew from the ground at a phenomenal speed choking them and dragging them down to the ground. The younglings then ran off, the men were unable to move and the dogs were also trapped.

It took another hour before mistress Vober's house came in to view. There were a few lights on and there were no guards at the gates.

They began speaking in whispers as they approached. The gate wasn't locked and it swung open making a rusty creaking sound. The house itself was quite large and they didn't know where to start. Nolon, suggested that the others wait for them outside, while Azul and himself would go in and try and find Dorian. They agreed and Nolon tried to open a smallish door that seemed to lead into the back of the house, but it was firmly locked. "I think we should skirt around to try and find a way in rather than breaking the door in," Nolon suggested. So, they wandered around the perimeter and found a swimming pool and just nearby was a groaning sound. Azul, rushed up to Dorian's wounded body that hung on a post, "Oh my god! What have they done to you?" Dorian was relieved to hear the voice of Azul and could only force out a few words of greeting. Nolon, untied his hands and Dorian slumped forward, they laid him down and Azul noticed all the pins that were stuck in him. She was horrified and began to pull them all out. Dorian, didn't feel the sting and jolted as mistress Vober's voice rang out, "What is the meaning of this?" she snapped at them. Azul, stood up and with much anger screamed at her, "*You're going to pay for this*!"

Miss Vober laughed and threw a *thread of dark matter* at Azul. It collided with her and the girl went down in agony. The *thread of dark matter* kept coming in a stream and intensified; the pain grew worse. "Oh, how I like torturing the unworthy," she said. Nolon, picked up a small rock and threw it at the terrible woman. It hit her in the face and she yelled in rage. This brought enough time for Azul to regain her composure and she raised her hand; a *flare of fire* burst toward the evil mistress and singed; burnt and set her hair alight. There was a brief moment when there was silence and miss Vober disappeared. "We've got to get out of here," Nolon said, "She will be back and probably with her guards. They lifted Dorian and carried him out to the front. They were slow going and a shimmering shield had sprung up around the grounds. When they reached the gate they couldn't leave for the barrier forbade them. Turning they saw about twelve men approaching with weapons and mistress Vober had a wand in her hand; it glowed with purple fire, crackling and spitting forth flames. They surrounded them and Azul dared not use magic, for some of the men had guns. Mistress Vober ordered them all to kneel and they did so. She motioned for one of the men to come near and he drew a sword. "We will teach these young fools a lesson," she said. "Execute them!" The man walked over to where one of the girls was trembling and sobbing. "No, not that one," and she pointed to Dorian, "Start with him." She had a great disliking to him and wanted his head severed for all the annoyances he had caused. The executioner raised his sword, but when it fell they had all disappeared. Mistress Vober upon realizing this let out an angry shout, "Where are they?"

Slonic, was relieved to see them all safe and well, except for Dorian's condition, as they materialized on the transportation pad. They were stunned for a bit and then when seeing Slonic they were overcome with gratitude.

The Lord of Death sat in the throne room cross legged upon the floor potting some plants he had purchased into a few selected pots which he had decorated himself when Faramel walked in. "We must retrieve the crown," the imp said. The lord was busy with tucking the roots into the soil and was half paying attention. Faramel then pressed a button for the television to come on and a picture of a alien dwarf came on, it was a programme called, The Angry Alien Dwarves of Pottenheim, a favourite of the lord, but he paid no notice. Faramel, couldn't help but feel sorry for him. He had lost his mind and even though in no pain he had lost the ability to be scary. The lord needed to have an aura of power and fear so as to get respect so people would behave. Without those qualities they would become complacent and would not revere him. "What flowers are those?" Faramel said pointing to a plant with a pink bell shaped flower. The lord looked at it and answered, "Oh, that is a *myculia* from the planet Gornia. Once it has grown it will sprout legs and run away to plant seeds in the ground before withering. "Interesting," Faramel said. They sat there for a while before Faramel thought that the lord was not up to getting the crown back so he went to see the masters, Quintok, Shein and Onis.

"The power of the crown is unique and therefore emits an energy that can be traceable," master Quintok said.

"Yes, yes. Just a quick spell from you should do the trick," master Onis said. Master Quintok rubbed his hands together as he thought of the appropriate spell to cast. It was a talent to be able to tailor a spell to a specific need and he was an expert in matters that required solving a problem. "Ani com duto," he said waving his wand. In his mind his vision took him out of the castle and along a road into the city until it entered the unholy church and settled upon the crown. "I now know where it is!" he exclaimed. "Not too far away. It is in the city. Within the confines of an old derelict church. He also saw the master of corruption and a few zombies. "We will need to be cautious though for there lurks evil upon our path."

They planned to retrieve the crown in the morning and would take two of the stone gargoyles for protection.

Zronisk, at this point was wearing the crown with the jewels in place and there was silence. "I can't hear anything," he said to Groni the goblin. He waited a while but still there was silence. Taking the crown off he inspected the jewels and they weren't shining. Groni, was flicking through an instruction booklet on making an immortal crown and came across a bit of information. "I think we need to charge up the gems," he said.

"What! It's one thing after another isn't it!" Zronisk slammed his fist down on the arm of his chair. "Well, how do we do that then?" he spat and then scratched his arm.

"Well, apparently we need to get the stone blessed by angel magic," Groni said with a pained expresssion.

Zronisk's rage was kindled, "What! And how are we supposed to do that? Can't we summon the spirit of darkness to descend into the jewels?"

"I don't think so. It is specific here that it must be done by the angels of light."

"Well we have to think of another way. It's just not the thing that I am going to do is it?"

Groni, winced and suggested that they pay some priest to do the job and then torture him afterwards just for the sake of his virtue. "No, no. We can't do that. It would be an insult to our god, except the torturing bit. Zronisk, collapsed on the floor and Groni said, "Are you okay?" The dark master of corruption groaned and said, "Do I look okay?"

Groni, smiled and said, "Are you suffering?"

Zronisk, managed a weak smile, "Yes, I am."

"Good," he said, "You can't always be in a good mood, you know it displeased our god if things always go well."

The corruptor raised himself to one knee and gasped for breath, "Something is happening to me, and I don't know what."

"Well, maybe you are dying. You know it is something to look forward to? To be united with the power of the dark one is a blessing."

Zronisk, let out a small laugh, "I am planning on living forever. But, my skin is scorched with some disease and I feel weak."

"Maybe your time had come. You know the dark one doesn't tolerate weaknesses."

He stood up, a little shakily and yelled for his followers in black robes. One appeared and he ordered him to go into the city and bring back a follower of virtue, he needed someone to torture to feel better, things just weren't going as planned.

At the *castle of fateful night* the others had returned without the gemstones and told of the followers of corruption who had cast spells on them and forced them to give over the jewels. They learned that the disease from the *crown of death* was tainting the land and many people were in pain. A selection of healers from the castle were sent out to ease the suffering and to bring relief to the ones inflicted. Though, the plague had no cure, with herbs and potions one could be kept alive a little longer. There was great sorrow across the land and many were dying.

When the morning came the masters set off down the road out of the castle's grounds and the bright sky was filled with birds. They had brought with them gargoyles that were over ten feet tall and made the earth shake under every footfall. The air was quiet around them as if the villagers from the outskirts of the city were not working on their fields today but the masters knew it was the disease that made the air silent because no one was around. It was the afternoon when they entered the city. There were beggars huddled in corners with flies buzzing around them. Also, the infected had to wear boards hung from their necks with a sign painted upon it declaring that they had the malaise. Sadness filled master Onis and people were watching as the gargoyles marched through.

Within an hour they had found the unholy church with the door hanging off its hinges. They walked in to the building with wands raised ready to cast a spell. Inside, it was gloomy and Morcego the bat flew in, it had been following the masters from the *castle of fateful night*. Zronisk, was awaiting them and had a plan. He was standing by the altar wearing the crown with Groni the goblin waiting in anticipation. "I think that that doesn't belong to you," master Shein said with a loud voice so it would carry over the distance. Zronisk, smiled a most self indulging smile and said, "I think you will find that it is on my head. Therefore, it is mine."

Master Quintok slowly walked towards him and said, "We will take it by force if necessary."

There were some stones with runes and dried blood in a triangle on the floor accompanied with markings of an evil nature and when the masters had entered the zone Zronisk, sprung the trap and dark magic surrounded the masters in a flash from the runes and symbols. A force field that wouldn't allow magic to be cast within its confines. They realized their vulnerability when they found that they couldn't move beyond a certain point. "Ah! It seems like I have you trapped!" Zronisk exclaimed in triumph and Groni let out a laugh, "See how easy it is to fool the virtuous." Zronisk agreed. The gargoyles stood still not able to form a connection with the masters who controlled them. Master Quintok said, "You may have us trapped but you are infected and will not last a week."

Zronisk, scratched his arm and said, "Oh, it's just a minor rash." The skin on his arm was withered and had spread up to his neck and around his back.

"I don't think so," master Onis said. "The *crown of death* has released a deadly disease and it has spread across the land."

"And I suppose you need the crown back to subdue it?" Groni said sardonically.

"Yes," master Quintok replied.

"Well, you really haven't got a choice have you?" Zronisk mused over their predicament. Morcego, the bat, flew up to the dark master and perched itself on his shoulder. Groni, ordered one of the other dark followers to go and get some fig juice and Zronisk added that he also brings a selection of crisps and chocolate. "It is going to be quite a night. You are going to be my source of entertainment," he smiled an uneven smile and contemplated in what way he could please himself with his new captives. There was a draft coming in through the door which irritated Groni and he set about trying to get the door back on its hinges, which took him a while. The door fell down after about half an hour and Groni resigned to the fact that it was going to be drafty. A dark follower entered carrying a woman on his shoulder. "Ah, so you've returned with a virtuous specimen?" the dark follower nodded and slumped the body on a bench. "Tie her up," he ordered and she was bound around the wrists. It wasn't long before she woke up and startled she began with a plea to be untied but Zronisk said, "There's no chance of that. You have been chosen."

"Chosen for what?" she asked.

"Oh, whatever crosses my mind," Zronisk said laughing. The woman began to get fearful and she glanced at the three masters within the zone. The dark master raised his wand and a scorpion snake appeared and slithered towards the restraining zone. It entered and attacked the masters. Master Shein gripped its sting and tried to snap it off and master Onis had his leg trapped in its jaw, he felt a sting as venom was pumped into him from the creature's fangs. Though master Quintok couldn't use magic he pulled out a small dagger from the side of his boot and stuck it in to the monster's eyes blinding it. The creature thrashed around and let go of master Onis. It fled from the zone leaving a trail of blood and slime. Somehow, it was able to enter and leave through the magical shield Zronisk had created. The dark master had watched on in excitement and Groni had cheered when the scorpion snake had gripped master Onis with its fangs. Things went quiet in the zone and master Shein knelt down to see to the fallen master. "I've been poisoned," he said and felt the effects of the venom coursing through his body. "I will only have a matter of minutes before I die," he said, knowing about the creature and its deadly poisonous venom. He reached for his herb pouch and pulled out a small paper bag with a variety of medicines. A tube of cream with tiny writing upon it was what he needed and he unscrewed the cap and squeezed some of it into the wound on his leg. "That should keep me alive for about an hour, then I will be no more," the immediate effect of the cream eased the pain. There was a round of applause from Groni as the creature vaporized into thin air. Zronisk then said, "Now that's added another dimension to the evening."

Master Shein bellowed out, "You're a coward! Why don't you fight with us on equal ground?"

"Well, it's more fun watching you suffer and die helplessly. There is something about the fact that you can do absolutely nothing about your circumstances and it is frankly quite humiliating for you, is it not?"

Master Quintok spoke, "I've seen your kind before. Feeding on fear and wallowing in the pleasure that it gives you to see others suffer. The Virtuous Creator will punish you."

"I don't think so! My dark Lord will out wit and overpower your puny god!"

"Our God is kind and merciful to those that follow his teachings, but justice will be given for those that defy his instructions and your dark god whom you serve will be brought to his knees and he will confess his iniquity, he will pay the price for his evil."

"I think you underestimate the power of my god," Zronisk said with an inflection. "He is servant to none. His power is eternal and he will not bow down to your God!" Zronisk, paced over to the stereo and pressed play on a tape recording of his choir that he had recorded. An unholy sound arose that chilled the bones of the masters. It was his zombie choir, at their best, though really dissonant and eerie. He left the room with Groni sitting on a stool with a cushion, as he went to get some more snacks from the store rooms. Where they keep the food was mostly empty and Zronisk ordered one of his speechless followers to go to get some sustenance from the local shops. He wrote down a shopping list and included things like, chocolate, apples, ice cream, cheese, pancakes, rice pudding, sausages, bread, sweets and vodka. The follower of corruption left with the slip of paper heading for the stores. While Groni was sitting there listening to the noise which Zronisk classed as music the woman who was tied noticed that master Quintok was trying to communicate with her. They managed to exchange words and she understood that to break the spell of the barrier that held the masters in the zone she needed to destroy the rune stones that were covered in blood. She looked around for something to do this and caught sight of Dorian's sword *steelfang* lodged under a bookcase. She wondered how she could get over to it and use it to free the masters when with a sigh Groni left the room to go and use the toilet. Realizing this was the perfect opportunity she rushed over to the sword, picked it up, and used it to smash the rune stones. There was a mild explosion and the woman flew in to the air landing a few feet away. Zronisk, at this point was just entering the room and to his horror master Onis cast a spell of *stillness* upon him. The dark master froze in mid step and toppled over hitting the ground in a puff of dust. The woman got to her feet and master Quintok thanked her for her assistance. He untied her and used the rope to bound Zronisk, then Groni peered around the doorway after hearing the explosion and was being cautious. He saw that the masters were free and instead of facing them went to get the zombie army. Master Shein took the crown and held it in his hands noticing the look of pure hatred on Zronisk's face. When the dark master had recovered from the spell he was angry and tried to summon a *lightning flash* to strike down master Onis, but the followers of the Virtuous Creator had tied a necklace of negation around his neck so casting magic was impossible for him. He cursed and spat on the floor threatening them with unspeakable torture and punishment. Master Shein laughed at this which infuriated the dark follower though he was helpless to do anything. They led him out of the building making their way back to the *castle of fateful night*. The woman thanked them and returned to her house and worried husband. Master Onis looked behind him and in the distance he could see the zombie army loping and limping behind, so they sent the gargoyles to deal with the problem.

The space craft which was heading for Skyworld sped easily through the darkness of space. Dorian was sleeping, curled up under a blanket, but the others were awake. They had healed him from his painful encounter with Miss Vober and his skin, which had been raw was now resembling its natural colour. The other young ones had decided to go back to Skyworld because their parents were nasty people. One boy said that he was constantly beaten at home and eventually sold into slavery. The others had similar stories and refused to go back to their families. So, Slonic, taking pity agreed to bring them back to Skyworld where they could begin their lives anew. Slonic, was most interested in hearing from Nolon and Azul about their adventures since they were parted and Slonic informed them that after they had run off from the dark follower and his zombie dog and minions, the *crimson fire gem* had been taken from him so he tried to hunt down the corruptor to regain it though had lost him in the city. They drank hot chocolate and nibbled on biscuits. All were grateful of Slonic's rescue and couldn't bear to think of what would have happened at the hands of mistress Vober, especially after how they had seen what had happened to Dorian in the short time he was with her.

Coruja, the owl, heard a knock on the door and a young boy appeared with a letter in his hand. He brought it over to where the owl had a book open and was reading from it until this distraction. He opened the letter and read it out: Greetings Coruja, I am informing you that the time has come for the *ceremony of fearsome divinity* as the current Lord of Death is no longer capable of his duties. I know of the prophecy and that the choice of the title is already in agreement with the council. Therefore, send word of when this has been done so that we can celebrate this momentous event with full confidence that the power that will be bestowed upon Dorian will be in accordance with every virtue that is needed for his role as sole Lord of Death of this realm. I send my warmest regards to you and will await your reply, signed by the Lord of Death 23rd realm. Coruja, blinked and the boy put the letter on the table and left the room. The owl had been observing Dorian since he had left for the planet Turgon and very much agreed with the prophecy. He felt that the boy had qualities that were essential for taking on the responsibilities as the Lord of Death and that though he was like any other boy, he had a meekness that would serve him well in his duties that he would be required to perform.

It was late in the day when the masters returned with the *crown of death* and Faramel was grateful to see it again. Master Onis was kept alive with magic spells from master Quintok and was taken to the healing rooms for the nurses there to save his life. He recovered within a couple of days after his blood was purified with a concentration of special flower petals that was in liquid form mixed with a small amount of sap from a local tree that grew in the castle grounds. All the plants, bushes and trees in the grounds were of some medical significance and the pupils in the castle were taught their value. The students studying herb lore were instructed in how to make pastes and elixirs from these useful plants and taught of their efficaciousness.

The space craft, under Slonic's control, landed in the grounds of the *castle of fateful night* and it was just becoming light with the first rays of dawn. They emerged from the space faring vehicle a little dazed for the air here was humid with the morning dew hanging off of plant leaves and shimmering in the early light. Azul, was glad to be back and so were the others. There were a few students around walking the grounds. It was advisable to get up early so that by the time the lessons began you had a clear head and had woken from the night's strange dreams. Dorian and Nolon went straight to their room and fell onto their beds grateful that they were out of harms way. Dorian, noticed the *uminin* plant that he was supposed to have nurtured, it was lifeless and withered; he thought to himself that he had failed a test, but he had had to leave this world in search of something much more important so he said to himself. Curled up in their beds it was not long before they were asleep. Slonic, took the homeless young ones to a small building were there were some beds and said that he would see them in the afternoon to talk about where they could settle on this world. They were given hope that a life here would be pleasant and that they would be free from torture and evil.

In the early afternoon when Dorian had woken up, and Nolon still lay there dreaming, he got dressed and headed down to the fountain in the gardens. Azul was there and she said, "Have you heard the rumours?"

"No, I have just woken up."

"Well, apparently there is going to be a new Lord of Death."

"What! How can that possibly be?" Dorian said in surprise.

"I think it has something to do with his madness. You know he has been acting quite strange of late. Apparently, the damage is irreversible and he has to abdicate."

"But who is going to take over?"

"All I know is that tonight, when we are all gathered together, the new Lord of Death will be announced from one of us!"

"One of us?"

"Yes, apparently someone has been chosen for the role of Lord of Death of this realm."

This left Dorian thinking who would be selected for this honour and Azul wanted to walk with him into the square where there were less people. They sat for a while and then Azul leant over to kiss Dorian and they were both engaged for a while before Dorian realized that his love for Azul was more than just friendship. They had a connection and his heart raced. "I've been meaning to do that for a while," she said.

When it was dark Faramel the imp went to see Dorian. He knocked on his door and when the boy replied he walked in and asked him if he would take a walk with him. The imp led Dorian to see Coruja the owl and the boy had no idea what for. Inside the room where the owl spent most of his time reading Dorian could tell that something was not quite as it seems for the three masters were there as well. "Dorian," master Quintok said. "We have some important news for you." Coruja looked up and blinked a few times. "I'll not beat around the bush. You have been chosen by prophecy to take over the role of the Lord of Death." Dorian, let out a gasp and said, "Why me?"

"Well, we don't always know why the prophecies choose certain people. But, we can be sure that it is the right choice," and master Quintok then let Onis speak.

"Our current lord, as you may well be aware, is not in his right state of mind and unfortunately it is irreversible while he is in this present form. So, therefore we need a new lord."

Master Shein then spoke saying, "The council of Mortis Divinus has required that we proceed with the *ceremony of fearsome divinity.* So, Dorian do you feel that you can accept this awesome responsibility?"

Dorian, thought for a while and said, "Maybe." But, his mind went to Azul and whether he would ever see her again.

"Well, it is going to be announced at one minute to midnight this evening," master Quintok then carried on saying, "It is a great honour to be chosen Dorian. Think on it."

He was then led to the gallery where they had paintings of the various Lords of Death that ruled over realms throughout the galaxies. Most of them still held the title and position of lord. His mind was swimming and he didn't know what to do so eventually he decided to go and take a walk around the grounds.

Whilst sitting underneath an old tree with triangular leaves Azul notices him and wanders over. "Hi," she says.

Dorian's mind was troubled for he didn't know what to say, after a brief pause he replied, "Hello, what have you been up to?"

Azul, smiled and said that she had been practicing the language of Hermosti. "And you?"

Dorian hesitated and decided to be frank, "I spoke to the masters. They want me to be the next Lord of Death."

Azul, let out a gasp of astonishment and said, "What did you say?"

"I said that I'd think about it."

She sat down beside him and small flowers from the tree fell around them in the slight breeze. "I would be honoured to take the position but what about us?"

Azul, had been thinking a lot about Dorian lately and their romance was just beginning to become something more. "I mean, if I was to live thousands of years, I think I might get lonely and I can't bear the thought of not being with you," Dorian's tone of voice held a sadness that Azul understood.

Azul, with an even tone said, "There is something about being mortal that is worthwhile. I mean, we would be together and maybe our love will last till we're old and grey, but if you were chosen to be the next Lord of Death there must be a reason. Something that you or I cannot comprehend."

Dorian, immediately defended his heart, "But, the way I feel about you. If I was to live for eternity, how could I with this burning love I feel for you. I would be unhappy and I don't think I could live with that."

They sat there in silence until Azul kissed Dorian on the cheek and said, "I will see you in the morning. I just need to see someone. I have an idea and it may help." She stood and walked away leaving Dorian to his thoughts. Azul, didn't mean to leave him in a state of anguish and despair but she thought that there might be a way where Dorian could be Lord of Death and she could be by his side as an immortal, as Lady Death. So, she went to see master Quintok.

At the sound of the bell chiming Azul knew that there was hope for herself and Dorian. She had read about the *ring of divine romance* and that a female could in fact be transformed into an immortal. It had been done before but not in this realm.

Master Quintok was sitting in the cool night air with a small fireball illuminating a book he was reading. He looked up as she neared him and smiled. He could tell she was going to ask a question or something so he spoke first, "Can I help you?"

Azul, sat down and let out her breath before confiding in the master her love and her fear of losing Dorian. "You know that to become immortal means sacrifice and duty don't you?" he said.

Azul, studied his face and responded meekly, "Yes. I don't want to lose him and I understand that my whole life will be different. But, it is something that I must do."

"You couldn't have had much time to think this through properly. There will be thirty days before the ceremony once it is announced tonight. Why don't you think on it and if you should choose to accept this marriage of immortality then I will give you the *ring of divine romance* the night before the *ceremony of fearsome divinity*."

Azul, couldn't help feeling that she had lost something. It was almost like having to wait in itself was a rejection of her love and sincerity. She walked away with tears welling up in her eyes, but was determined that when the thirty days were passed that she would take the ring and be a part of the ceremony to live forever with Dorian.

Tentatively, she walked back to where Dorian was sitting under the tree whose flowers were arbitrarily falling and was pleased to see him sitting there in thought. "Hi," she said with a hint of sadness.

"Where have you been?" Dorian asked.

She explains to him about the *ring of divine romance* and Dorian feels that there may be hope for them both to be together. But, at the same time he is sad, "I don't know what living forever would be like. I don't know if it will become unbearable or if I will get bored, I just don't know if I am able to deal with it..."

Azul, didn't know either but said, "We could see sunsets from other worlds. We would be free and fearless to walk the night and we would visit the spirits of the departing and say kind words of reassurance. We would be able to walk hand in hand across deserts and climb mountains without fatigue. We would be together and our romance will be legendary." Dorian smiled at this and thought about having Azul by his side as his Lady. "Maybe it would work if we both became immortal. After all we would have each other." They sat in silence for a while and Azul plucked the small flowers from Dorian's hair which had fallen from the tree. After a little while they stood and walked to where Nolon was sitting playing music. The night drew on until all the inhabitants of the castle were gathered in the main square awaiting the announcement to be spoken at one minute to midnight.

The masters were assembled on a platform in the square and Coruja the owl was seated on a cushion. The Lord of Death was nowhere to be found for he was swimming in the sea on planet Dargoni. When it reached one minute to midnight the bell from the chapel rang out once every ten seconds. Master Shein spoke, "Tonight the name of the new Lord of Death will be announced. It is a sacred and honourable position. To be selected for this duty one must possess certain qualities and no man may choose whose title this may fall upon, but instead the person can only be named through the prophecies, for which Coruja is the author." The bells began to toll as it had reached midnight in a quick succession. "The privileged title belongs to... Dorian Bluefeather!"
There erupted a great cheering and master Onis brought Dorian to the platform and said, "You may say some words."
He felt nervous but the need to say something was important, "I will say that it is a great blessing to be chosen to be the Lord of Death and I promise to rule wisely and that there will be no unfairness in my judgements," he stopped there and the people began another round of applause. Dorian stepped down and took Azul's hand; they walked through the crowd amid cheers and celebrations. There were tables of cakes and pitchers of flavoured fruit drinks but Dorian's head was swimming so they both walked to the fountain and sat there. "I was going to say something about you wanting to become Lady Death but it didn't seem right."
Azul, smiled and said, "We will announce it at another time, but for now they know that you are the one to be crowned Lord."

Master Quintok, knocked on the door of Nolon and Dorian's sleeping quarters, it was a week before the ceremony. Dorian, who had been lying on his bed studying the language of Hermosti, placed the book aside and said, "Come in." The master gently opened the door and peered round. He had *steelfang* in his hand and Dorian was surprised for he had thought his magical sword was lost for good. "Here, I return this to you," the master said. Dorian, took the sword and unsheathed it. The blade was clean and there were no chips of scratches on it. It felt good to hold and its weight was balanced. "Thank you," he said, but words weren't enough to express his gratitude for the sword had been in his family for generations.

The day was almost upon them, when Dorian would be crowned Lord of Death and the transformation will be complete. Azul, found master Quintok, after he had just led a class on turning elements into useful weapons, in a room full of old books that were piled from floor to ceiling. "Ah, Azul. How can I help." She felt almost offended that it didn't bring to mind that she was here for the *ring of divine romance* and that her previous request was not seen as sincere, 'How could he forget?' she asked herself. He turned and before she could speak he said, "So, I presume that you still want to go ahead with the unity of immortality?"

Azul, managed to raise a smile and said, "Yes. The ceremony is tomorrow and you promised me the ring. Is this still possible?"

"Oh, of course!" he stepped down from a raised platform where he had been arranging some heavy tomes. "Come with me," he said strolling out and across the courtyard. She followed and was led to see Coruja the owl. The owl was eating some fried meat and soya chunks and it took a few minutes before he was finished. Master Quintok requested the *ring of divine romance* and Coruja scribbled a note for Azul to read: *What is the most important reason that you want the ring?*

Azul, read this and then said, "Well, I want to be with Dorian for the rest of my life."

Coruja, then scratched another question on paper: *Why is this important to you?*

She thought about the book of Everlasting Truths and had read somewhere that love was the highest attainment of virtue and that without it nothing is of value, so she said, "My love for him is my highest form of sacrifice. For him I would give anything including my mortal life."

Coruja, seemed satisfied and flew out of the window. Azul, seemed a bit worried that she had said something wrong but the master said, "We will wait for a few minutes, he shouldn't be too long."

The owl flew onto the roof of the building of decay where no one has access to and clawed a small stone lid open. Inside was the *ring of divine romance*. He clutched it in his claws and then flew back to the master and Azul.

When he had flown back into the room he dropped the ring into the girl's open hand and master Quintok said, "There you have it! You are one step closer to immortality."

She looked a little uncertain about the consequences what the ring means and the significance that it held. Master Quintok then said, "Don't worry I have sent for your parents for I knew that you were not going to refuse the notion that the ring would be the only way you could be with Dorian."

Azul, smiled, feeling that the master hadn't doubted her love for Dorian.

The Lord of Death returned after Faramel had located his postion by tracking down the *mino ring* the lord wore. He had informed the lord that the crown had been recovered and that the *ceremony of fearsome divinity* was to take place the next day in the presence of night. The lord sighed and said, "I suppose it is time that the bug divorced the moth and we can be a happy family again." Faramel, knew that the lord wasn't in any pain but felt that it was not good for him to be so influenced by insanity because you couldn't really have a conversation with him. He felt sad, but was looking forward to seeing the lord transformed into the mortal he once was when the ceremony was complete. They were soon at the *castle of fateful night* and the lord decided to do some gardening.

The night had come for the *ceremony of fearsome divinity* and Dorian knew Azul was a little doubtful of the whole thing but to be binded together for eternity was something they both wanted. They stood in a clearing, with jasmine bushes a sweet scent in the air, in the *forest of guardian spirits* and the masters of the *castle of fateful night* with a host of others that were to be witnesses of this momentous occasion were present. Haroman, Brina, Martiv and Tinina were excited about Dorian's prospect of becoming the 5th Lord of Death of this realm. Azul's family were also there and her mother wept with uncertainty of her only daughter and that she would live for millenia; joy was also present. Slonic stood next to Ormapruviel the female elf whose beauty was remarkable. Coruja, the owl was perched on a branch of a tree and looked on in anticipation. The musicians began to play their instruments and a choir of skilful singers began their summoning of the angelic host. A stirring in the forest could be felt and the air began to swirl as several spiritual angels appeared with shining raiment and soft voices as they hovered, their feet not quite touching the ground. The Lord of Death knelt down in front of them and a most beautiful angel with long curls of hair lifted the crown from his head and light shot out of the gems, each ray a different colour creating a rainbow of immense brilliance. A chord of sound emanated from the crown which was in tune with the instruments the players were evoking and a humming surrounded them all accompanied with a circle of deep darkness. Master Onis motioned for Dorian and Azul to step in to the *circle of darkest night* and they did so. Dorian felt a lightness in his heart and Azul clasped his hand and kept close to him. The angel with the crown then said, "Hold up your hand Azul."

Tentatively, Azul lifted her hand with the *ring of divine romance* on her finger. The myriad of rainbow light from the crown coursed toward the stone in the ring and entered it; she began to feel radiant and blissful until the power surge ceased. Then the angel said to Dorian, "Kneel."

Dorian knelt and the crown was placed on his head. It shrunk to his size and the bony skeletal figure of death began to undo and strips of light mingled with darknesses spiralled around his skeletal frame until a young man was remaining in a sleep. The power then, spinning around, directed itself into the crown and Dorian shuddered; as the immense energy that seeped into him began its transforming work. At this point the jewels emanated a sparkling arc of many colours which went into the *ring of divine romance* on Azul's finger, transforming her also. Music was all they could hear as the angels began their *song of immortal life*. Moments seem to fade in to years as their life flashed through their minds and Azul and Dorian could see the universe as their minds travelled around the galaxy and soared around planets. It seemed like this was their domain, they belonged and would rule over the fate of many of the worlds they were now seeing. Dorian, could hear hushes as the music died down and he felt his mind was alight. He stood tall; looking over to Azul he saw that she was Lady Death. A skeleton in appearance but what radiated from her was a beauty he found mild yet gentle and her mind instantly glowing with love. He took her hand and kissed it. Then the angel spoke, "The *jewel of universal sadness* is still frail, but it will in time draw in the disease which is scourging the land and then your power of mind knowing will be complete and the virus will be confined once again." There arose then a great cheering as the spectators roared in enthusiasm and respect. Haroman, came over to his son that stood over nine foot tall and patted him on the arm saying, "You will always be my son, even if you out live me by thousands of years."

Dorian's fire eyes shimmered a blue sparkle, "And you will always be my father. The memory will always be with me."

Tinina, ran up to Dorian and hugged him as best as she could with tears in her eyes, "I love you," she said.

"I know," he replied and grateful for the affection she was showing.

There was a great celebration that lasted to the dawn. Rykin, who was the previous Lord of Death was taken to the healing rooms to recover. He was murmuring and sweating quite a lot, but Dorian knew that he would recover and that his mental state would be healthy. Faramel, sat in a chair next to the bed waiting for him to awake but knew it might be a few days, even still he would wait.

The next day Dorian was explained his duties by Coruja the owl who would scribble down things of importance like people he had to meet that would be alliances and worlds to visit. Azul, was also present, as Lady Death, and she mostly had to accompany the lord on visits and her duties were mainly paper work but the most crucial thing she had to do was to maintain the power of the jewels in the *crown of death*.

Both the Lord and Lady had to sign a paper agreeing to uphold the virtues of the Creator and to serve him and the people to the utmost of their abilities. Once this was signed Coruja spelt out another note: You must be wondering?

"Wondering what?" the lord said.

The owl wrote some more words: How you escaped the sharks that time you were thrown to your certain death.

The lord thought about it. *Yes, it had seemed strange that the creatures were completely docile and unwilling to tear me to shreds with their sharp teeth*. Then Coruja pointed a wing at the lord's wrist. The lord looked down at the necklace, of the black shark's tooth, that he had strapped to his wrist and said, "Oh, that's why!"

Coruja, motioned for him to pick up another note he had just etched, it said: A gift from the Creator.

The disease from the *crown of death* was retreating from the lands and people were beginning to see plants thrive and the immediate deaths had ceased. Indeed the *universal jewel of sadness* was becoming brighter.

Zronisk, was kept in a lower chamber in the castle grounds. He had been the subject of a variety of tests. The results revealed that he was corrupt in every darkness, there were no specks of virtue, they were all destroyed. This, led to the masters choosing one option that was preferable to his death. The result of a serum that could be injected into his blood would eventually, within a matter of days, lead to the break down of memory so that all of Zronisk's magical knowledge would be forgotten. Though, this also had an effect on language capabilities it would mean that he wouldn't be able to cast any spells. The dose was administered, it was the only option. He

117

would become almost like his zombies. He would have to learn to read and write again, and within the *castle of fateful night* he might even be able to nurture his divine sparks and follow the Creator, that was their hope. The followers of dark corruption, that were under his spells, were without a master and they left Skyworld to seek a world where they could continue their unholy religion.

When Rykin had awoken, Faramel was there. It took a few moments for Rykin to acknowledge what had happened. "You're back in the land of the living," the imp said. The young man Rykin, managed a brief smile, "So I am," he said. "How long has it been?" he enquired.

"Oh, thousands of years."

He looked sad for he had no known family to see or anyone who he knew from the days he was previously mortal. Faramel, knew this would be a concern and said, "Don't worry... You can make new friends," he said, "And, you now have the opportunity to find a wife and have children of your own."

Rykin, thought about something he hadn't even contemplated in such a long time. "I guess you're right. And, right now I could do with something to eat." He swung back the bed sheet and dressed in clothes that had been laid aside for him on a chair. Faramel, then said, "I think you will find that food tastes a lot better now you have a tongue!" They both laughed as they made their way into the sunny courtyard.

The Lord and Lady stood beside Juiz as he explained his duty and service to the Lord of Death. The 5th Lord of Death of the realm sent the rat on his first mission to judge an evil person. It was a matter of hours before the rat was knocking on a door. He waited for a while until he heard someone curse that their servant was not around and, "I'll just get it myself shall I," referring to answering the door. It swung open and mistress Vober stood there towering over the rat Juiz. "Miss Vober?" he asked. "Yes, what is it!"

The rat raised his hand with the card with the emblem of the *castle of fateful night*, the owl reading a book, "*Preordained by death*," he said and there was a flash of light...

The End.

Errol Edward França Hewitt

Milton Keynes UK
Ingram Content Group UK Ltd.
UKHW041313210924
448622UK00001B/19

9 781783 821204